Praise for Find...g ... ...

"*Finding Your Forever Body* offers a practical yet transformative approach to help readers develop an entirely new mindset, along with a new set of tools. This book is a must-read for anyone who's been on the diet cycle for many exhausting years!"

MARCI SHIMOFF, #1 *New York Times* bestselling author of *Chicken Soup for the Woman's Soul* and *Happy for No Reason*

"Before you try another diet, I highly recommend you read this book. Kimberley's guide helps to take away the overwhelm, frustration and self-criticism that we face by living in a diet- and 'perfection'-obsessed culture. Supportive and informative, her passion for nutrition and 'body love' shines through every page."

JANET BRAY ATTWOOD, *New York Times* bestselling author of *The Passion Test*

"I love that *Finding Your Forever Body* provides a kinder, gentler way for those who struggle with food and body image. Using her own personal story as an example, Kimberley provides a guide for the reader that's inspirational, compassionate, and life-changing."

TERRI BRITT, former Miss USA, award-winning author of *The Enlightened Mom* and founder of *Women Leaders of Love*

May '20

Jenn,

Keep shining
your gorgeous
gifts with the
world! ♡

K xo

Finding
Your
Forever
Body

KIMBERLEY RECORD

A 10-Step Guide to
Breaking the Diet Cycle for Good

Finding Your Forever Body

WINGPOWER
PUBLISHING

WingPower Publishing
Campbell River BC Canada
KimberleyRecord.com

Cataloguing data available from Library and Archives Canada
ISBN 978-0-9958673-0-7 (paperback)
ISBN 978-0-9958673-1-4 (ebook)

Produced by Page Two
www.pagetwostrategies.com
Cover design by Peter Cocking and Michelle Clement
Cover photo: Shutterstock
Interior design by Peter Cocking
Printed and bound in Canada

17 18 19 20 21 5 4 3 2 1

This book is dedicated to my daughter, Eve,
whose loving spirit, generous smiles, and crazy-fun sense of
humor remind me every day of what true beauty is.

Contents

· · · · ·

Introduction

. . . .

> *"It does not matter how slowly*
> *you go as long as you do not stop."*
> CONFUCIUS

Your Forever Body

· · · · ·

HAVE YOU BEEN struggling for months or even years to find your ideal diet solution?

Are you frustrated with all the options and information overload out there?

Have you become so diet-reliant that you feel like you're doing something wrong when you're not following a diet's guidelines or at least monitoring what you're eating?

I was struggling, frustrated, and diet-reliant for a long time, too. In fact, for almost 15 years, I was so disconnected from my body that I wouldn't know what or how much to eat without a diet plan. If you can relate to this feeling, you're not alone.

But what if, rather than watching what you eat, you were simply nurturing and nourishing your body with what it needs at that moment?

I'm not talking about satisfying a craving; I'm talking about *really getting to know what your body needs to function at its best* (otherwise known as **intuitive eating**). This crucial skill, I've learned, makes maintaining a healthy lifestyle so much easier, and much more enjoyable. The freedom from diets that I'd personally craved for years became possible at last because I finally learned to tune into and respond to my body's needs. And this is a skill that we *all* have the capacity to master, as long as we have the commitment to fine-tuning our self-awareness, building our knowledge, and making our self-care a priority, for good.

But typically, it's the "for good" part that scares a lot of people. This is why diets rarely succeed over the long term. Most people can give up their favorite ("unhealthy") foods for a short period of time in order to achieve a goal. But that sacrifice is usually short-lived because sacrifice equals pain; and as humans, we subconsciously do everything we can to avoid pain—we are literally programmed that way.

So how do we maintain a healthy body for good if we can't give anything up for good?

For the sake of our well-being and our self-confidence, we need to first commit time to shifting our mindset before we approach *any* new program or lifestyle change. We need to start looking *inside of ourselves* for the answers.

Enter the Forever Body...

My Forever Body is what I've affectionately come to call my body after overcoming years of food and body image struggles: it's the body I'll willingly put a bikini on any time of year, no matter what. This is what I want for you too.

A Forever Body is not a bikini or beach body, or a wedding body, or a New Year's resolution body, but rather a body that you can be proud to nurture and nourish for life.

It's a body that consistently improves over time in health, function, and appearance as you add each new positive, health-supportive habit to your life.

It's a body that may be ten, twenty, or more pounds away from your "ideal weight" but that speaks to you intuitively about what size and weight is the most supportive for your optimally functioning body and mind, at that time.

It's a body that's easy to maintain because it feels good to do things that support it—and when you're not doing them, it feels very uncomfortable, even painful.

It's a body that makes you still feel healthy and energetic 10, 20, 40, 60 years from now, no matter what's going on in your life—not one that gets "punished" with each new season, diet, job, relationship, or any life stress.

· ·

NOTE: An important aspect of a Forever Body mindset is the language we use to describe our food and lifestyle habits. Intentionally, I use "supportive" and "unsupportive," rather than "good/healthy" or "bad/unhealthy." Here's why:

Good/Bad and **Healthy/Unhealthy** are used when external influences motivate our choices, and I feel this takes away our free will. ("I should/shouldn't eat that.")

Supportive/Unsupportive are used when internal influences motivate us. We've personally determined what supports our goals, and we're empowered to make our own choices. ("I will/won't eat that.")

"Healthy" foods or habits may be identical to "supportive" ones, but the way we refer to them can create positive mindset and behavior shifts. So going forward, I encourage you to always speak from a place of empowerment.

It's a body that, when in balance, will reward you with energy, vitality, and an *inner glow* you will be proud to shine, no matter your size. (When it's out of balance, you will feel like crap and be constantly searching for how to feel better. You may even indulge in temporary "pleasure fixes," which all leave you feeling worse after overindulging.)

The most important thing to know, trust, and deeply believe is that your Forever Body is *yours*. *You* get to set the standards and determine the path that's right for you. Therefore, I'm not going to tell you what and how much to eat. That is up to *you* to discover.

Sound like too much work? Trust me, it's not—once you master how to really listen to your body, it's very simple, and I'm going to show you how to develop the crucial skills you need to do this. And to have fun with it!

Breaking the Diet Cycle

This is not a diet book. I'm *not* going to teach you how to lose weight in a short time frame by restricting calories, entire food groups, or pleasure from your daily intake. The pain and exhaustion I've personally experienced with dieting have caused me to run from diets and cringe at the word "calorie." From my teenage years until I was 30, my body image ruled my life: I was obsessed with calorie counting, fad dieting, and weighing myself. I could never fully enjoy the experience of eating, or living joyfully for that matter.

Thankfully, over recent years, through research and education, as well as personal reflection and discovery, I've been able to gain clarity about my true definition of health—physically, emotionally, and spiritually. This has ultimately led me to achieve my Forever Body.

Although my journey is continuously expanding and my quest for knowledge is always deepening, I feel compelled to share what I've learned thus far because I see that what I've been through is not unique. So many others, especially women, are dealing with similar emotional battles with food, weight, and body image, at the expense of real joy, freedom, and self-love. And the solution is not just about food.

Nutrition is a huge part of health, yes—but there is a deeper foundation to be established before any long-term results can be realized and maintained. This is the premise of my ten-step process.

Like me, you *can* stop obsessing over food and the number on the scale, so that you can start living your life free from dieting for good. *At the same time*, you can enjoy the process of achieving your healthiest body yet, because this also isn't about going to the opposite extreme and "giving up" on your body.

If you are carrying extra pounds, I promise you will release as many as your body needs to feel its best, as long as you apply the principles I'm sharing here and *lose your diet mentality for good*. This is probably the hardest thing you will have to do, because, as a culture, dieting has become our go-to whenever we want to make a physical change. Releasing the weight will become *easy* once you've officially let go of the idea that you need to diet in order to do so.

Here's a critical truth that will hopefully help you to do this:

Most weight-loss programs (that is, *diets*) are designed to set us up for failure.

Don't believe me? Just look at the stats. Well-publicized studies have shown that 95 percent of dieters who lose weight will gain it back, and then some, within five years.[1] Not exactly encouraging results to conclude that diets work, or that the companies that create them even have our best interests in mind.

When dieters regain weight, they continue to pump money into products and systems that will help them to lose it again. In North America, this cycle has made weight loss a 55-billion-dollar industry.[2]

But that's not the worst part. What's even more sad than the financial toll this takes on us is the toll it takes on our self-esteem, our happiness, and ultimately our ability to realize our full potential because there's always an underlying unfulfilled goal. Speaking entirely from experience here!

There are four main problems with the diet mentality:

1. We've been sold on a set of unrealistic standards[3] that keep us feeling "not good enough" no matter how we look or how much we weigh, which seems to have us constantly focused on trying to live up to them through some program, product, or system.

    Statistics show that 91 percent of women are unhappy with their bodies and resort to dieting as a means to correct whatever it is they think needs fixing.[4]

    Please let that statistic sink in a moment: 91 percent of women are on a vicious, seemingly never-ending diet cycle!

    Given that the percentage of women who are obese or overweight is much less than 91 percent,[5] obsessive dieting and body image concerns are not just problems that overweight or obese people deal with.

2. We've been sold on the idea that the only way to really lose the weight we want to lose, or to achieve the body we want (that is, the one we've been sold), is to diet—which leads us to feel as though we're doing something wrong when we're not dieting.

   It's not all our fault that we've developed this mentality—marketers are skilled at tapping into our insecurities and appealing to our pain points to sell more of their company's products. Eighty-five percent of diet product consumers are female,[6] so it's no surprise that ads are mostly aimed at us. But it's not really the marketers' fault, either.

   The interesting thing is that when a diet doesn't work, it's not necessarily the products, services, or programs that are to blame; in fact, many of them can be very effective, useful, and supportive tools that we can use on our journey toward better health.

   But the industry now gives us a seemingly endless stream of options, some of them conflicting, which offers us an easy "out" if something doesn't work for us. When we can blame something *outside of ourselves* (like a product or program) for our inability to lose weight or to sustain the weight loss we did achieve, we can easily abandon our efforts and move on to the next thing—but not before we revert to our old, familiar, unsupportive habits first.

   This is the (dreaded) diet cycle, and it needs to stop.

3. We've internalized the idea that dieting is good for us. But the truth is that dieting is a form of **disordered eating**,[7] and can negatively impact our physical, mental, and emotional health tremendously. Though different from

an eating disorder and not necessarily life-threatening, disordered eating is any form of controlled or restricted eating in which we're disconnected from our body's natural cues and needs—as is the case with dieting—and it's also a real problem and a much more widespread one.

4. The fourth—and possibly most harmful—idea is that losing weight is a direct path to self-confidence, self-worth, and self-acceptance. Though it may be unspoken, this is a belief that many women grasp onto (as I once did), because we're influenced by messages everywhere that solidify it. Maybe this rings true for you:

"Once I lose the weight (or get the six-pack or fit into that dress), *then* I'll be happy and move forward confidently in my life (work, business, relationships, etc.)."

The problem I see so often is that so many people— women especially—*put life on hold* until they've reached a point of being happy with their bodies, which is usually associated with a number on the scale, dress tag, or tape measure. That's what I did for so many years.

We typically believe that once we get to that point, then we'll have the mental and emotional freedom to put our energy into bigger, more important things in life: we want to reach our ideal weight, so we can then be happy,

• •

By the way, marketers love that we think this way. It's this mindset that keeps us spending our hard-earned money on their products and programs, instead of other possible investments. I don't even want to think about how many vacations or personal development programs I could have enjoyed with the money I've spent trying to unsuccessfully "fix" my body!

and then we'll start living the life we want. Or, put another way, that's when we'll *feel worthy* of the life we want.

And yet being tied to a diet is the exact opposite of freedom.

The diet industry, in general, does not promote the lessons I'm sharing with you because

1. they don't cater to a quick-fix approach; and
2. if everyone had their Forever Body and no longer felt the need to lose weight, diets would become obsolete. Not good for business.

But I *want* diets to become obsolete. I *want* you to have your Forever Body, so that you can shift your attention from obsessing over food and your body weight to the things that give you passion, purpose, and joy.

I *want* you to overcome your self-limiting beliefs about your body and overall image, so that you can unleash your true greatness out into the world.

I *want* you to feel confident throwing on a damn swimsuit any time of year, so that you can get in the water and *play*!

I want all of that, and more, for you, which is why I'm so glad you've found this book.

What if . . .

What if you could take your life off "hold" and build a body and life that you love at the same time?

What if you could feel totally at ease and confident in your body *now*—so that you can start living the life you want, right away, while at the same time start building a healthier, stronger body?

What if you could start setting your own standards and metrics to measure your progress and success, rather than relying on outside sources?

What if you could stop obsessing over food and the scale, so that you can use your precious energy on things that give you *joy*?

What if you could *create a life that you love* by embracing, nurturing, and nourishing your unique body—not by trying to fix, punish, or deprive it of pleasure? And what if, by doing this, you could actually build a body that you'll love for the rest of your life, without ever dieting again?

Well, I'm here to tell you that you can. That's a Forever Body. And it's already yours to access, right now.

Sound too good to be true?

If I hadn't done it myself, I may have thought so, too. Though it took me a looooong time—over 15 years—I did manage to break through my old, limiting beliefs. In the process, I came to the realization that the only way I've ever achieved what I really wanted in my life, including a healthy, vibrant body, was by treating my body as my friend and ally—*not* as the enemy holding me back.

Dieting never was, and never will be, the answer to long-term health and happiness.

Finding Your Own "Perfect" Solution

I hear *so* many women—even those who look to be within their normal healthy weight range—talk about the need to "lose weight," "watch what they eat," or "start dieting again," and then allow this to be an ongoing distraction. I was there, so I know the feeling well.

I remember being in that exact same state of mind. I often kept my thoughts to myself, though; I didn't talk about my feelings about my weight because I was embarrassed that I hadn't yet figured it all out for myself, that I hadn't yet found my perfect solution to keep my weight from constantly fluctuating.

I hid my feelings behind a pretense of self-confidence, deflecting attention from my body and relying instead on other ambitions and superficial "successes" for approval. But, behind the mask, I was miserable. The extent to which I allowed my worth to be tied to my image started to affect *all* areas of my life, including my relationships, my love and sex life, my social life, my work and finances, and my ability to *play*.

I was so busy trying to live up to external standards that I had become disconnected from *who* I really was and would literally cry myself to sleep some nights. I was lost; and I don't feel that my story is unique. I suspect that if you're reading this right now, you might be able to relate to these feelings, at least on some level.

However, I believe the combination of tools and principles that I've applied to finally achieve a body—and life—that I love *is* unique. I've achieved a long-term sustainable body weight and size that's "perfect" for me, because it supports me in being the fullest expression of my authentic self.

I also believe that if more women had these tools to discover their own "perfect" solution, we could see that statistic of 91 percent decrease dramatically.

The Rewards of a Forever Body Mindset

A Forever Body is for everybody. Whether you are currently dealing with the prospect of losing five pounds, a hundred pounds, or more, I believe that everyone can benefit from developing a Forever Body mindset *now*.

When you do, before you know it people will start asking what you've been doing—and you may not even be able to give them a specific answer because it's happened as if you weren't looking. You will grow older, but you won't age. You will become healthier, fitter, more energetic with each passing day—and each time you see an old friend, they will notice. These are not empty promises; these are all very possible outcomes available to you, if you're committed to the process.

Sharing my experience and acquired knowledge with you has become my passion, my mission, and my purpose. I want to help you fall in love with your body and with yourself; to separate your size from your self-worth; and to enjoy the process of nourishing yourself the way you are physiologically designed to do. This is why I've taken the time to

The Dalai Lama says that "the world will be saved by the Western woman."[8] Yet, when 91 percent of women are allowing themselves to be held back and distracted by body insecurities, what could the world be missing out on? With a new approach to body love, I believe, comes the potential for greater impact, whether it's on the whole world or just one person's world.

Where would *you* start to invest your energy with this newfound emotional freedom?

reflect on and summarize the lessons I've learned through-out my own journey into a simple process.

I'd like to say upfront that these steps *require time, patience, and a commitment to consistent improvement.* They require you to take responsibility for your health and take over the reins from the diet industry. This process is not a quick-fix approach that will guarantee overnight results, but if you take the time to truly follow these steps, I believe they will help free you from ever having to embark on another "diet" again.

They are designed to help you experience a lifetime of true *body love*, starting today.

A quick note on eating disorders and other medical conditions: this book is in no way designed to replace the advice of a medical practitioner. I do believe, however, that a positive shift in mind-set can strongly contribute to the healing process of any dis-ease. Therefore, this book may serve as a useful tool that you can add to your tool belt as you work through your healing journey— even if you just learn and adopt one new positive way of thinking.

"The only journey is the one within."
RAINER MARIA RILKE

Why Would You Listen to *Me*?

∙ ∙ ∙ ∙ ∙

THOUGH I HAVE over ten years' experience as a Registered Holistic Nutritionist (RHN)[9] and professional Health Coach, I'm also here speaking to you as a woman who knows what it feels like to be completely out of tune with—and even hating—her body. Prior to my career in wellness and nutrition, I'd been part of the 91 percent for over 15 years—a time during which an obsession with food, the scale, and achieving "perfection" ruled my life. Some people have told me I can't possibly understand what it's like to constantly feel I'm "not good enough," because I clearly don't have a weight problem and never really have. But I do understand, and I can relate—very vividly.

I think it's important to address this upfront because I'm not overweight, and I've never truly had a "weight problem" per se (though I *have* been a few sizes bigger than I am currently). Nor have I ever experienced a full-on eating disorder. But I *do* know what it feels like to be *extremely* unhappy with my body and my weight—and to be caught in the vicious diet cycle.

I know what it feels like to step on the scale first thing in the morning and have the number it displays determine how happy and confident I'll be for the rest of the day. I know what it feels like to meticulously measure out my portions, listen to my stomach grumble all day, and walk around in a starvation-induced brain fog. I know what it feels like to wear baggy clothes to hide my thighs and to walk into a room hoping no one notices me because I'm having a "fat" day. And I know what it feels like to see pictures of myself and tear myself down for every little physical "imperfection" I want to change. (I started doing that when I was three!)

Therefore, even though I've never been technically overweight, I'm very familiar with the internal struggle that comes with desperately wanting to lose weight and the impact this can have on *all areas of life*. And that's ultimately what this book—and the diet cycle—are all about.

Whether we are overweight or not, it's fundamentally all the same: if you feel bad about your body, it's not the number that's the problem; it's what you're telling yourself about the *meaning* of that number that's the real underlying problem.

It's not about the number—it's entirely about the mindset.

While I *could* write a book on nutrition, fitness, and healthy weight loss, and teach you how to get the body of your dreams, that wouldn't address the underlying problem—which wouldn't fulfill on the "for good" part of my promise to you. Therefore, I'm writing to you instead as a woman who's been in your shoes and sharing how I finally began to embrace, nurture, and nourish my body with ease (and without diets!), so that you can accelerate your journey to get to this same place.

To help solidify your confidence in me as someone who understands what you may be going through, here's a little more insight into my personal diet cycle:

"My Thighs Are Fat"

I was three years old the first time I uttered these words.

You may be surprised to hear how young I was when my own body-image issues began. But this is not an exaggeration. My mom still tells me to this day: "You're probably the only three-year-old ever to complain of having fat thighs! And I don't know where you got that from—you never heard it from me."

And I believe her, because it was certainly not a case of repeating what I'd heard.

Although I was generally healthy and active as a kid, I had the belief from a very young age that my body should be different and "better," because I compared myself to other children—in particular, to my slightly older, yet much tinier stepsister. She had skinny legs and arms, and I had a larger body type with "more meat on my bones," as the saying goes. Every time I saw a picture of us together, I noticed—and internalized—the differences between us.

My First Diet

I was 11 years old when I tried my first diet, straight out of a teen fashion magazine.

Even though, by this age, I'd sprouted up taller and become leaner, I still believed that I was bigger than I was supposed to be and that I should be dieting to change and improve my body.

I had watched my mom go on diets for years, so I just knew that dieting was the way to ensure that I wouldn't get fat. Of course the magazines constantly confirmed this: I loved flipping through their pages, chock-full of beauty and "healthy diet" tips, and I was "inspired" by the models they showcased. I decided that the closer I resembled them, the more confident and accepted I would feel.

This was not only my first experience with dieting and feeling the pain of starving from severe calorie restriction, but it was also my first—and definitely not my last—experience with bingeing.

At that age, I'd already begun to realize there was something wrong with this process since it was so uncomfortable and frankly scary to be "out of control" with bingeing—but I thought that if all the adults I knew were doing it, there must be something to this dieting thing. I was determined to figure it all out.

My "Typical" Teenage Struggle

Rather than attempting another diet at that age, I just began to "manage" what I was eating, based on my magazine-acquired nutrition knowledge. For about five years, I consumed little more than black coffee for breakfast and, for lunch, always two rice cakes with peanut butter and a Granny Smith apple. I would eat these slowly while watching my lean, athletic friends eat hearty sandwiches, poutine, burgers, and whatever else they wanted.

I rarely ate with my family for dinner, because I'd get home after school ravenous, raid the cupboards, and no longer be hungry for a prepared meal. I was also resistant to their "meat and potatoes" lifestyle, which my magazines had informed me was *definitely not* the way to go if you wanted to be thin. Instead, after school, I filled up on loads of dry cereal, fruits and veggies, and low-fat yogurt. Since "low fat" was the trend at the time, I avoided anything fatty like the plague—and usually consumed excess amounts of low-fat foods.

When I went out with my friends on weekends, I would order water and salad while they continued to enjoy their feasts. They all played sports, but since I was always hungrier after exercise and was worried about overeating, I never took to any sporting activity myself. I blamed my lack of athletic coordination and ability for my lack of interest, and I managed my physique strictly with my diet.

The Modeling Years

My "figure management" (that is, food-restriction) system seemed to be working for me—although it was probably more true that my young and efficient body was working rather than my "diet" itself. At age 15, I decided to enter a modeling contest. I was chosen as a finalist to participate in a local fashion show—and I loved it! So I quickly took up modeling with an agency in my small town.

It felt *amazing* to have an activity that I enjoyed outside of school. I loved dressing up in new clothes, swimsuits, and lingerie. I loved getting my hair and makeup done. I loved doing photo shoots. Even though I didn't get paid for any of it (and, in fact, had to spend my own money on photo shoots and courses), I still loved the feeling of getting outside of my comfort zone and overcoming my shyness in front of a crowd and a camera. What a wonderful, confidence-building experience modeling had started out to be.

My Turning Point—for the Worse

After a couple of years of strutting my stuff on local catwalks, I got an opportunity to meet with a reputable modeling agency in the big city, for a "go-see." These interviews allow agents to see your body and face in person, and to determine whether or not you're a fit for their needs.

I enlisted the chauffeur services of my stepdad for the day, dressed in my most flattering clothes, applied my makeup to perfection, and showed up excitedly for my appointment. And in under 15 minutes, my self-esteem was ripped to shreds.

At 137 pounds and 5′8½″ tall, I was told that in order to be successful, I would have to lose 12 pounds, grow by half an inch, and get braces for my less-than-perfect bottom teeth. And this feedback wasn't "sandwiched" with anything positive.

This was my moment of transformation from a teenager who was slowly working to overcome her insecurities about her body by flaunting it unapologetically onstage, into one who felt completely unacceptable, even ashamed, because of it.

My stepdad stood by me the whole time and afterward tried to cheer me up the best way he knew how: "Screw 'em, let's get you some French fries!" he said as we stopped for lunch on the way home.

So appreciative of his support, I devoured a plate of fries and returned home for some crying and quiet reflection. I decided quite promptly that modeling wasn't for me anymore—I had no idea how I would ever lose 12 pounds, except by starving myself, and I knew I couldn't do that. And if I couldn't lose the weight, I couldn't be successful, so what was the point?

And So Began My Diet Cycle . . .

I thought that quitting modeling would solve my problem of not feeling good enough about how I looked. But it was, in fact, just the beginning of a bigger problem.

Since I no longer had my fun extracurricular activity, I began to focus on my social life, which involved a lot more partying. I took up drinking and (cigarette- and pot-) smoking on the weekends—things I probably would have managed to avoid had I felt more self-confident in my social settings. Although it was all mild, nonaddictive behavior, my indulgence in these vices contrasted starkly with the "healthy" food regimen I tried to stick to during the week, as the partying was almost always accompanied by fast food and other junk.

Yet I watched the scale diligently—and daily. Even though I *thought* I'd rejected the idea of ever reaching 125 pounds, 137 pounds now seemed a completely unacceptable number. I didn't want to starve myself, but I soon realized that was the only way I could make up for my weekend habits without gaining weight. I would go about my weekdays trying to stay busy so that I wouldn't think about food, hoping there wasn't too much quiet reading time in my classes, when others would be able to hear my grumbling stomach. I never felt energetic or even happy; I now realize that was probably in large part due to nutrient deficiency.

My negative body image had slowly taken over my life, and although, thankfully, I never developed a full-on eating disorder, the consequences of my "weight management" habits—bingeing and severe restriction—on my health, energy, mood, and self-esteem would literally take years to repair.

My Personal French Paradox

Restricting and bingeing became a regular routine for me throughout the rest of my high school and university years, until I had an opportunity in my last semester of university to participate in an exchange program. For four months I lived and studied in Rouen, France, a beautiful city north of Paris.

Though I was bursting out of my skin with excitement, I was also feeling another emotion that was equally pronounced: fear. Not fear of being in a different country, meeting new people, and studying at a different school— those were all thrilling prospects for me. What I really feared was one of the big cultural adjustments I would need to face: eating what the French eat.

I wasn't just afraid of the French Diet; I was petrified of it! Loads of white bread, pastries, cheese, fatty meats. What the hell would I eat?

I was relieved when I found some of my staple foods in the local *supermarché*. *This way*, I thought, *I can still party and indulge in high-calorie drinks, and make up for it by eating cereal and carrots all week.*

As I settled into my life as an expatriate, I very quickly witnessed the French Paradox all around me: the locals ate fatty, decadent foods (and enjoyed every bite!) and they drank wine daily, yet they were incredibly lean, in general. Naturally, most of us exchange students began to adopt the lifestyle—it was hard not to—and many of us started to lean out, too.

When I eventually gave up my resistance to adopting a different way of being and living, I started spending less time in my room by myself eating carrots dipped in dry oats (yes, I really did this) and more time with my friends in the *salle à manger* eating five-course meals together. Eating became less of a stressful duty and more of an enjoyable experience.

I was seriously confused whenever I took the time to think about it, though. What I'd been doing to feel lean and light went against everything I had read and thought I knew. White bread, pastries, and cheese definitely didn't fall into the acceptable food guidelines I'd committed to memory and followed diligently prior to this trip. But I was loving the feeling of being okay with it and having my body follow suit, so I didn't question it.

I eventually came to see my leaner body as a side effect of having the time of my life (with less time to obsess). When my repatriation to Canada arrived, I tried to bring this feeling and mentality back with me, but that didn't exactly have the result I was hoping for.

My Repatriation into the Standard (North) American Diet (aka SAD Diet)

I couldn't wait to weigh in when I returned home. I didn't want to become scale-obsessed again, but I did want to have a number to associate with the way I was feeling. I figured I was "strong" enough to resist the temptation to weigh myself more often. After all, *not* seeing the number daily was part of my formula for finally feeling okay with, and in, my body.

I was delighted to see the scale said 130 pounds: just five pounds away from my "ideal" weight and the closest I'd ever been as an adult! I even resolved at this point to officially change my goal weight to 130 pounds because of how good I felt. The problem was, I had no idea how to incorporate my new French lifestyle into my North American life, which now included graduating from university and getting a full-time job. The fun, travel, and party life had ended.

Since I'd allowed myself to actually develop a love of food (mostly) without guilt and wanted to make sure I maintained this healthier mentality, I started off by not depriving myself at all: I ate whatever I wanted, whenever I wanted. But I quickly packed on the pounds—about 15 to be exact.

I was confused again. Wasn't this what had been working so well for me? There went my theory that I could eat whatever I wanted, as long as I enjoyed and savored it the way the French did. (What I didn't realize at the time was that *quality* of food made a big difference, something the French are known for!)

Panicked, I quickly went back to the only thing I knew that worked for me at home: dieting.

The Ongoing Search

For years after that, I continued the search for my "perfect" diet, reading countless books about new eating and exercise programs—and I was trying a new one, it seemed, every new Monday, new season, and new year. I felt like I was constantly on a diet. Probably because I was.

I was also more scale-obsessed than ever. It didn't help that 140 pounds was "heavy," according to popular opinion and the media. By this time, I was hovering around the 148-pound mark, so the unrealistic standards made me believe I was now extremely overweight. Despite my dieting efforts and my regular scale gazing, I seemed to be constantly watching the number go up and it was starting to affect all areas of my life.

My Turning Point—for the Better

Fast-forward to age 29. I was miserable in my job, unhappy in my year-old marriage, and wrought with anxiety most days. I'd not only subscribed to external standards about my appearance but in pretty much *all* areas of my life—which had led me to a point where I felt completely out of place in my body, my relationship, my home, my job, and even my family. Having always been a relatively upbeat and positive person, I was surprised to find myself in a place I never thought I would be, and at such a young age: I was depressed. My whole life was out of alignment with who I was and what I wanted, and it had become extremely painful.

The pain was physical, as well as emotional. My diet cycle and food obsession had started to wreak havoc on my body: my digestion, immune system, and energy levels were the worst I'd ever experienced.

I knew I had to start healing my relationship with food in order to regain my health, and so I determined that I needed to learn more about it. For the first time in my life, I made a choice that felt truly my own: I left my suffocating, stifling corporate job to pursue studies in natural (holistic) nutrition. And that decision caused a domino effect in all the other areas of my life, as I began to come out of the dark hole of obsessive dieting and measuring my self-worth by my size.

Once I started making changes that matched my true passions and desires, my life—and my body—began to transform. This marked the beginning of a stage in my life when I finally felt that I was setting, and living by, my own standards. Though it involved some big initial and extremely difficult decisions, like leaving my marriage and moving across the country, it also allowed me to begin attracting new people, situations, and opportunities that were more aligned with me. And as the other areas of my life began to heal, so did my relationship with food and my body.

After this initial transformation, I learned that having a strong foundation of self-awareness, self-worth, and self-care doesn't necessarily make life easier (there have been many ups and downs since!), but it certainly helps to create a greater sense of empowerment for pulling through whatever life tosses my way. And what a difference that makes.

Body Love Starts with Mom

The biggest mental shift for me happened seven years ago, when I became a *mom* to a beautiful little girl—my daughter, Eve. Despite all the positive steps I'd taken to develop a healthy self-image, I knew I still had some work to do because it scared the crap out of me that she might follow in my footsteps.

Though I don't blame my own mom for my body-image struggles and conditioning—she had been conditioned, too—now that I knew better, I felt I had a huge responsibility to become a body-positive role model for my daughter.

I desperately wanted to prevent her from going through the same painful negative self-talk I'd experienced through my earlier struggles. I knew that my little girl would be watching my every move, and I was hell-bent on raising her with a strong sense of self-worth and high self-esteem. And it had to start with me.

Today

Today, at age 41, I'm proud to say with all confidence that *I love my body*. All 140-ish pounds of it. I'm also proud to say that I don't know what the exact number is—and that 98 percent of the behavior and attitude I model to Eve is indeed giving her a healthy foundation of self-esteem and true body love, inside and out. Here are some things we do every day to build on this foundation:

• We talk about what we love about our bodies—never about what needs fixing.

- We focus on our strengths, progress, and staying true to ourselves—not on being perfect.
- We make a conscious effort to nurture and nourish ourselves and our bodies—without depriving them of pleasure.
- We move our bodies everyday because it feels good—not because we need to burn off or "earn" our food.
- We celebrate our differences and uniqueness—instead of judging them.

Of course, there's always that clingy 2 percent that still needs "managing," but the most important thing to me is that, *at any moment, any day of the year,* I'll throw on a swimsuit to get in the water and play with her!

Such a *huge* shift emotionally from where I was ten years ago.

Mentally, there have been major shifts, too:

- I *never* step on the scale—or even have the urge to.
- I haven't picked up a diet book in over ten years.
- I feel sexy naked.
- I am no longer petrified of fat.
- I delight in eating dessert every day.
- I enjoy moderate amounts of red wine and coffee regularly, and I relish the occasional night out with friends for beer and French fries (guilt-free!)

Physically, things have also shifted as a result:

- My clothes always fit.
- I eat when I'm hungry and I stop when I'm full.
- I eat what I want, when I want (which has a totally different meaning to me today than it did back when I returned from France).

- I enjoy generous servings of most things that I eat so that I'm satisfied.
- I rarely have a "craving."
- I'm in the best physical shape of my life, even though, as a general rule, I work out for *no longer than 30 to 40 minutes, no more than five days a week.*

As a bonus, I also seem to have developed an immune system of steel, and I have even more energy than I ever had in my teens and twenties. This has allowed me to take on physical and mental challenges that I could only have imagined doing back then—running a marathon and writing this book, to name a couple.

Both my body *and* my life have transformed as a result of some simple (though not easy) changes in the way I relate to food and my body—particularly my weight. These mental and emotional shifts have shaped new beliefs, behaviors, and habits that have allowed me to become the body-confident role model that I want to be for my daughter.

But it's been a hell of a journey to get here.

I know the frustrations, and the ups and downs, involved in getting to this place of inner peace and self-acceptance.

• •

Eating an entire avocado in one sitting… spreading *real* butter on a freshly baked whole-grain muffin… enjoying the occasional crispy skin off a deliciously seasoned roasted chicken… These are all things I couldn't even imagine doing for at least 15 years of my life because I was terrified of fatty foods. But, today, I can delight in doing any of these whenever the urge strikes—without guilt and without consequence. What changes could a Forever Body mindset bring in *your* life?

You name the emotion, I've probably had it along the way—and probably still do from time to time!

Though my journey may—and most likely does—differ from yours, the lessons I've learned can be applied to any situation. Your journey may be more or less dramatic or traumatic, and it may take more or less time to travel than mine, but that's not the focus here. We're all on our own journeys, and it's important to remember that our bodies are as unique as our stories: no two are exactly the same.

It's time to start acknowledging this and to embrace yours.

Each day is a new opportunity to continue the journey in a new direction, to choose a new path. I'm here to help make the navigation a little easier for you. Consider this guide as your body-love GPS. You will ultimately find your own way, and follow your own path, but the process of doing this is always a little easier when you have a road map to help you get you where you want to be.

It's also easier once you become aware of the *roadblocks* in your way, which is why it's important to first address what may have kept you from succeeding at dieting (and/or keeping weight off) in the past: the reasons I believe that most diets are setting you up for failure.

In the next section, Part 1: A Common Problem, I'll be sharing with you the top seven reasons that diets don't work, as well as why you shouldn't be so quick to blame your willpower. I'll also provide you with nutrition information that's crucial for you to know before embarking on any new change to your diet or lifestyle. Then, in Part 2: A Unique Solution, I'll guide you through my ten-step process for breaking the diet cycle for good and for enjoying the journey toward permanent change, starting right now.

1

A Common Problem

. . . .

*"Don't let the science of nutrition
interfere with the art of eating."*

NICK HALL

The Top Seven Reasons Diets Don't Work

· · · · ·

FROM MY 15 years of experience with unsuccessful diet-ing and ten years of studies and professional experience as a health coach and nutritionist, I've identified seven key reasons why I believe most diets are setting us up for fail-ure—whether they do so on purpose or inadvertently.

The reason I hear most often for failure to stick to a diet is a lack of willpower. But you won't find this in my top seven. I firmly believe that this is never the real reason; there is so much more to maintaining a healthy body weight than simply willpower. Although *taking responsibility* for our own health is critical to be able to sustain results, *blaming* our-selves or our lack of willpower for a lack of success is not helpful and can, in fact, be very harmful.

It's Not Your Lack of Willpower

"I just don't have the willpower" is a truly destructive belief, and here's why: our beliefs project themselves on all areas of our lives—our health, our work, our relationships, and even our finances. So when we believe that we lack the willpower to stick to a diet and successfully lose weight, this can not only cause us to give up on our health goals, but it can also lead to feelings of inadequacy and dissatisfaction in many other areas of our lives.

Over the past several years, it's become one of my biggest pet peeves to hear the words "If only I had the willpower to…" Many people talk about willpower like it's a magical gift that only a select number of special people have been blessed with!

I get so annoyed by these words because

1. it's an all-too familiar sentiment that reminds me of my old thinking patterns, and
2. I know that *everyone* has this "magical willpower."

Most people are just missing what's needed to activate its magic: a *true commitment to their desired outcome* (which consists of knowing exactly *what* they want and *why* they want it).

Willpower is just another word for self-control, discipline, determination, resolution … and it's impossible to maintain it without a clear vision of and commitment to the desired outcome. It's *commitment* that motivates us to stay on track toward our goals, not willpower.

We don't often say "If only I had the commitment to…" because this implies we're taking personal responsibility for not doing the things we know to do in order to get where we (claim we) want to go. It's much easier to blame our lack of willpower, which many imply is something that's out of our control (you know, because we haven't been blessed with it from birth).

Here's what's important to acknowledge: commitment, and therefore willpower, is quite simply a personal choice, and it is entirely within our control. Yes, we get to *choose* what we commit to! But I'd be willing to bet that most people don't consciously choose their own weight-loss goals. Most often, our goals (especially those pertaining to our bodies) are determined on a subconscious level by social influences, medical and professional opinions, and/or the media, which is possibly the worst influence of all.[10]

When you are properly equipped with the right tools to solidify *your* commitment, you may never need to worry about a lack of willpower again. When true commitment is present, willpower follows easily. (I'll help you develop those tools in Part 2.)

I guarantee that you already have the willpower to succeed at whatever it is that you're striving for, in any area of your life—and you've always had it. If you walk and talk, your willpower was at work even as an infant to learn these crucial life skills. We *all* have it in us; we just need to be clear on *exactly what we want and why we want it*, which we'll get into in your ten steps.

So now that we've cleared up this misunderstanding about willpower, let's take a look at the real reasons that diets don't work.

The *Real* Reasons Diets Don't Work

As you read, please keep in mind that the word "diet," in its originally intended meaning, simply refers to the food that we eat; and there are many reputable experts who can help you learn some basic and extremely supportive and effective approaches to healthy eating (aka developing a healthy diet). For the sake of clarity, I'm not necessarily referring to all nutrition plans that exist out there.

The "diets" I'm writing about here are mainly those commercial diets that currently make up the 55-billion-dollar weight-loss industry:[11] the generally unsustainable, popular, fad approaches that have prompted the mis-use of the word, promising "proven" weight loss in a specified (usually short) amount of time.

The fact is that anyone can restrict their calories for a short time and lose weight. But how many people can maintain their healthy weight, within five pounds, for over five years—or even forever? The answer is: *only* those who choose a non-diet approach.

Here are the top seven reasons why:

Diet-Fail Reason #1:
They can't give you what you're really looking for.
The smiling faces in the "after" pictures of diet ads would have us believe that happiness, our ultimate (perceived) goal, can be achieved through weight loss. Unfortunately, we've been misled—and we've been misleading ourselves by believing this.

I hate to be the one to break it to you, but losing weight *won't* make you happy. In fact, it's been widely supported[12] that this common belief leads many people to extreme disappointment when they reach their goal weight and find that they're not any happier as a result. You may have even experienced this yourself.

I can speak from personal experience: when my weight was at its all-time lowest—about a year after I had my baby, and breastfeeding had literally depleted my body—there was so much stress in my life that celebrating a newfound thigh gap couldn't make up for any of it!

Even though, by that point in my journey, I'd been living a holistic lifestyle and eating intuitively with natural nutrition for about five years, I realized that I was still just as invested in *looking* good as I was in *feeling* good. During that time when I was really thin and also really unhappy, it finally dawned on me that there was more to this whole happiness thing and that the quest for a "perfect" body never was the right route to take for achieving it.

Since then, I've made my happiness the biggest priority in my life. I've learned that it's not even a goal itself (that is, it's not something to be achieved). Instead, it's a fundamental element of reaching any goal in life—and it's an inherent state available to every single one of us, right at this moment. I attribute everything I have today—including a lean, healthy, and energetic body that I'm proud of—to the discovery of how to be happy without first changing a single thing about my life or my body.

When I reflect on my Personal French Paradox, I see that it gave me an early taste of this feeling that I continued to crave ever since. As soon as I gave up my fear of the fatty foods that were part of the local cuisine, embraced the joy of eating, mindfully ate moderate portions, and enjoyed good company and conversation along with the meal, my clothes started to fit better and even became loose. I had no access to a scale, so I really had no idea at the time how that translated into pounds, but I felt lighter, my digestion was more efficient, and I had a lot more energy to stay up till 4 a.m. at the club.

Unfortunately, I wasted over half of my exciting, four-month French adventure stressing about food and my body. But, even though it took a while for me to fully allow myself to integrate with the culture and the environment, this shift still had an amazing impact on me: I felt a total sense of freedom when I wasn't being constantly weighed down by the stress of figuring out what and how much I should eat.

My happiness—fueled by the excitement of doing something I love—had freed me from my food and body obsession, and, in the end, it resulted in improvements not only to my physical health but to my mental and emotional health, too.

So, if you've been waiting to hit that number—on the scale, the dress tag, or the tape measure—before you allow yourself to start being truly happy, to live your life fully, to cease obsessing over your body, I urge you to stop waiting. The number isn't really the goal; the smiling face is. Happy is. And you can decide to be happy now—before you even lose an inch. How? Keep reading, beautiful! I'm going to show you the way...

Diet-Fail Reason #2:
Most diets aren't customized for *you*.

No two people are alike in genetic makeup; therefore, everyone will respond differently to nutrition plans and even lifestyles.[13] For example, some thrive on high protein, while others do on vegetarian diets; some thrive on intense cardiovascular activity, while others find that more moderate, gentle activity works best for them.

When high numbers of people try the same diet, it's likely that it will only work for a small portion of these people.

Granted, there may be common guidelines that work for many—such as avoiding wheat and gluten—but that likely has more to do with the refining and processing of the food itself, rather than its nutritional biochemical effect on the body. If everyone ate only the unrefined, whole-food variety of the grain, in much more moderate portions, it wouldn't have the same impact on inflammation and weight gain in the body. (Only a small percentage of the population is actually allergic to wheat.)

No diet plan can tell you exactly what *your* body needs, in what proportions—only you can discover that. The good news is that we're naturally designed to do this; the bad news is that we've allowed ourselves to be reprogrammed with a plethora of expert, often conflicting advice that makes up the diet industry. So much for relying on our bodies' intuition. It's no wonder that, at any one time, 108 million people in the U.S. alone are on a diet.[14]

It's also worth noting here that your current weight is *not* just a result of your daily food intake, and therefore it cannot be modified (permanently) with diet alone. There are other factors at play, which are also unique to you: your stress, your activity level, your relationships, your social life, your sleep, and your environment at work and at home.

Nutrition—which is actually what you *absorb*, not just what you eat, and there's a big difference—is the largest factor, and I stand firmly behind the notion that it's responsible for about 80 percent of your state of health. But it's not the only one. So if you haven't yet achieved the results you're looking for, it's imperative to also examine the other 20 percent and seek solutions that are right for your unique situation—and of course, use your nutrition solution as a support tool as you address those other factors. Don't worry, I'll be guiding you through this in Part 2!

Diet-Fail Reason #3:
The start date is the most exciting part, and the rest is just hard.

Personally, I've always loved the excitement of starting something new, the thrill of a new challenge. I'm curious, I crave adventure—and what better way to add some spice to life than to embark on a new program for improving my health! That's how I used to think, anyway.

But what I realized, after declaring many "fresh starts," is that the preparation and start date were the most exciting. What usually followed after the start date was that I would either become bored, overwhelmed, and demotivated, or I would recognize that I hadn't completely *mentally prepared* for permanent change—and I would easily get derailed when I couldn't perfectly stick to a diet plan.

To prepare, I'd typically spend days before my start date consuming extra amounts of the foods that I wouldn't be allowed, clearing out my fridge and cupboards of all restricted foods, and even packing on a few extra pounds to get super motivated before Monday (my habitual start date). But usually, as soon as Tuesday or Wednesday came around, I would start searching for another solution that might not be as hard. (I realize that most people probably last longer than this on a diet, but I'm sure many of you can relate.)

Quickly, I'd go back on the hunt for my "perfect" diet, or sometimes even switch on my "everything in moderation" mentality—which was never effective for very long, and you'll see why in the next chapter.

It wasn't until I finally gave up my "all or nothing" mentality—either "all in" a diet, or in binge and prep-mode—that my life and body began to really change. I've learned that eating a health-supportive diet doesn't have to be hard at all and can even be quite enjoyable.

This has also taken a lot of pressure off New Year's Day and Mondays. Aren't they already stressful enough?

Diet-Fail Reason #4:
They encourage us to change *multiple* habits all at once—and habits are difficult to change!

The fact is, most diets aren't designed to allow us to develop new habits in a way that supports permanent change. Most of them are structured to have you change *many* things all at once.

So much research has been done on the process of habit changing, and it's quite an elaborate process. It requires a keen awareness of your current habits and triggers, as well as a deliberate commitment, and subsequent conscious effort, to replace old habits with new, equally rewarding ones.[15] It can take months to change just *one* habit permanently.

When we try to change so many things in our lives at one time, it can not only overwhelm us, but it evades the proven process for permanent change. Inevitably, we create too much discomfort, which leads us to easily slip back into our old lifestyle and eating habits because of their pleasurable familiarity—despite the fact that the comfort they provide is usually only temporary.

Given that the two main human motivators are pain and pleasure—and that, in general, changing habits can be a painful process to go through—for permanent change to occur, we need to first acknowledge that either

- the effects of the old habit are *more painful,* or
- the desired effects of the new habit are *more pleasurable than the pain of changing!*

If either of those statements isn't the case, we're not likely to permanently change our habits until one of them is true.[16]

Our habits are what shape our lives, and a change in habits can literally change our lives, so we first need to get crystal clear about how we want our lives to transform, while also ensuring that the outcome matches our values and beliefs.

Anyone who's ever achieved and maintained a healthy body has simply been successful at developing habits that support them in doing so. It isn't any more complicated than that. Although the process of changing habits is simple, it's not easy and most often requires support. Most diets never address this underlying foundational work, and therefore they are setting us up for failure.

Diet-Fail Reason #5:
Your body is "protecting" you from losing weight.

When we lose weight too fast, as is typical on most diets, there are several biological reactions in the body that start kicking in to keep us safe and alive. The body is smart and keeps track of all changes, ensuring that nothing gets out of balance for too long. When we start "wasting away," it will quickly get to work on reestablishing homeostasis—even if we aren't literally wasting away, that's how the body interprets quick weight loss.

Our physiology plays a significant role in whether or not we can successfully achieve a permanently healthy weight. When we take a dieting approach, which is usually restrictive rather than nourishing, we may experience quick weight loss, but the body's protective mechanisms will soon kick in. This can lead to frustrating results that have nothing to do with your willpower, or lack thereof.

According to a study published in 2011 by the *American Journal of Physiology,* we all have what's known as a "steady state" weight, which is a range determined by a number of factors, including biology, environment, and behavior (all influenced largely by genetics).[17] The body interprets this steady state as the range it needs to stay in to ensure it stays alive and well—even if this steady state is in a clinically overweight or obese range. It's the range it's been familiar with for most of its existence; it knows it well and doesn't wish to deviate from it.

How does the body ensure we stay in this steady state range? Well, it's now a well-known fact that metabolic rate decreases to preserve energy when the body believes that it's starving—a common reaction to severe caloric restriction. When metabolism decreases, our muscles become much more efficient and don't need as much energy (calories) to function. Therefore, unless we lower our caloric intake *even more* to accommodate this reduced energy requirement—which is very difficult to do, especially if we're already feeling deprived—we can easily regain weight.

But research has now found that there's even more to the equation than just decreased metabolism. Here are some other of the most noteworthy factors.

For starters, our hormones are also part of the picture, and one that plays perhaps the most critical role is **leptin**—produced by our fat cells, it's the hormone responsible for signaling our brain when we're full. When we diet,

- our fat cells shrink too quickly,
- our leptin levels drop,
- our brain receives a signal that our energy stores (fat) have fallen too low, and
- this leads us to overeat, or eat when we're not really hungry, in order to bring our body out of its energy-depleted state.

There are more chain reactions that start happening in the brain too, including

- increased activity in the part of the brain that experiences pleasure when eating, which then increases desire for the immediate "reward" that comes with eating, and

• •

DID YOU KNOW? When we lose weight and body fat, we never lose fat cells. They only decrease in size.[18] The one exception to this is liposuction, where fat cells are removed (which comes with its own set of risks and complications, including kidney and heart problems,[19] so I definitely don't endorse this!). There are actually only a few times in our lives when our number of fat cells change. They increase in the womb during the third trimester, before we're born (which is totally out of our control), and we also gain fat cells during puberty, pregnancy,[20] and anytime in adulthood when a significant amount of weight is gained.

- decreased activity in the part of the brain involved with restrained eating, which then decreases our ability to consciously make more supportive choices.

When I think back to my first diet at age 11, I can see how all of these functions kicked in very quickly. I remember lasting about four days on the calorie-restricted diet of celery, rice cakes, and canned tuna. I can recall getting home from school on that fourth day and, almost as though I was possessed and out of control, running directly to the kitchen and cleaning out the cupboards. Cookies, Pop-Tarts, cereal—whatever carbohydrate I could get my hands on, I ate. And I couldn't stop.

My body and my brain were literally starving of nutrients and had finally taken control over my "willpower." They were trying to get as much energy as possible into my system, as quickly as possible. And I didn't keep off the weight I'd lost for very long.

So, you can start to see the bigger picture of why dieting, and losing weight with "proven," "quick" strategies, can really cause more harm than good and will almost always lead to weight regain, because that's how we're biologically designed to react. An approach that allows the body's steady state weight to change gradually over time is more likely to prevent these physiological reactions and better support sustained results.

Diet-Fail Reason #6:
Most diets emphasize what you *can't* eat.

Diets generally encourage us to eliminate particular foods or entire food groups, often using a cold-turkey approach—and have you noticed how much *more* you want those foods when you know you can't have them? There are two underlying reasons why the cold-turkey approach is detrimental to our efforts and ultimate success at making permanent changes.

The first is our human tendency to avoid pain. Perceived deprivation—especially of foods that we may have turned to for comfort—is painful, period. Even if we're depriving ourselves of a food that we don't eat in excess or even all the time, we begin to crave it more as soon as we know we can't have it.

As humans, we're innately drawn to experience pleasure and to avoid pain. So, subconsciously, our minds will do anything to prevent us from experiencing pain (deprivation)—and we can consciously fight it for only so long. We might do really well restricting forbidden foods/drinks for a couple of weeks, even months, but at some point we will break down and want to consume copious amounts of those things we've been depriving ourselves of. Then, we'll feel crappy about ourselves, and our capabilities, believing that we aren't strong enough or that we don't have the willpower. This can have a devastating effect on our self-esteem and on our resolve to make permanent changes.

The second underlying reason, which also relates to the subconscious mind, is that, biochemically, our brains are designed to help us seek out the things that we're focused on, good or bad. The part of the brain responsible for this is called the **Reticular Activating System** (RAS),[21] also known as the gateway from the conscious to the unconscious mind.

It's the part of the brain that allows us to filter out all the unnecessary information that we're exposed to every day, in order to avoid overwhelm and keep us focused. It does this *subconsciously*, following the *conscious* guidelines we give it.

In other words, what we're consciously focused on—in this case, what *not* to eat—is what the RAS will subconsciously seek.

This is part of the magic behind the **Law of Attraction,**[22] which states that whatever you focus on expands. In other words, the more attention you give something—positively or negatively—the more you will naturally attract it into your life or environment.

So, if you've ever had the experience of trying to eliminate something from your diet and then wanting that "restricted" food *more than ever*, this is what's happened. If you're focusing on what you can't eat, your subconscious mind will be your worst enemy, while it's thinking it's your best friend. You may start to notice those particular "forbidden" foods everywhere you look, which will make avoidance even more difficult and those foods even more tempting for you.

Diet-Fail Reason #7:

They put most of the emphasis on the quantity of food that you eat (usually through calorie management), but this math is seriously outdated.

Burning more calories than you consume is simply not enough anymore—at least not for a long-term, sustainable plan. Back when our food was not so processed, refined, and genetically and/or chemically altered, the equation of "calories in < calories out" was much more relevant. Today, a calorie is not just a calorie. Food *quality* is more significant than ever.

"Eat less, move more" is an overly simplistic and outdated philosophy, and one that leads many people to feel worse about themselves when they can't just do something "so simple."

A lack of energy and/or motivation to follow through on the things we know to do can usually be traced back to our nutrition (what we absorb from our food), which is a direct result of the quality of food we're eating—*not* the quantity. Simply counting calories, carbs, or fat grams can leave us with a *huge* gap in the nutrients that we require to keep our energy, mood, and motivation high.

Food producers and marketers are also relying on our diet failure for their profit, and they are working tirelessly to ensure that we don't succeed (see the next chapter "Why Our Food Is Stronger Than Our Willpower").

If you are eating refined/processed food (also known as "ultra-processed food"), you are susceptible to food manu- facturing practices that are sabotaging your health and your weight-loss efforts,[23] no matter how "calorie controlled" they are. If you're still consuming even moderate amounts of these foods, your body's physiological responses to them are literally stronger than your willpower could ever be.

Our bodies will do anything to maintain homeostasis, and these foods inevitably disrupt this balance. Reactions such as increased cravings, inflammation, and blood sugar imbalances are common as our bodies work to reestablish homeostasis—reactions that don't bode well for self-control. Our food, therefore, is indeed stronger than our willpower.

In fact, addressing these physiological responses is so critical to breaking the diet cycle for good that it's worth diving into even deeper.

*"Tell me what you eat, and I will
tell you who you are."*

JEAN ANTHELME BRILLAT-SAVARIN

Why Our Food Is Stronger
Than Our Willpower

· · · · ·

"OUR FOOD IS *not* our grandparents' food" is one of the most memorable statements I heard while studying natural nutrition. And it's so true! What does it mean? Increasingly, food manufacturers, for the most part, have become more concerned about their profits than our health. This wasn't the same reality for our grandparents growing up.

The food industry has grown exponentially over the past few decades—and to our detriment, unfortunately. As the population and average body size have increased, so too has the demand for food. One of the negative effects of this has been a reduction in quality—both of the processed/prepared/packaged foods and the raw ingredients (meat, dairy, produce, and even our herbs and spices are affected). So we can't simply eat the way our grandparents or parents ate and expect to maintain the same level of health as they could back then. We're just not getting the same nutrition that once existed in our food supply.

Rather than rant about food manufacturing and what it's doing to our collective health, I've instead provided more detailed information in a free online *Nutrition Resource,* which you can access by visiting www.FindingYourForever Body.com/Resources. The purpose of this section is to draw attention to the fact that *what* we eat has become just as or more important than *how much* we eat—particularly when it comes to achieving and maintaining a healthy, lean, and vibrant body for good.

The important thing to note here is that the quality of food that you eat may be in large part to blame for your apparent lack of willpower and/or inability to achieve a healthy weight or size, despite your best intentions and efforts.

The following are prime examples of common manufacturing practices that do *not* have our best interests in mind:

- The refining of ingredients to reduce production cost and increase product shelf life.
- The addition of addictive ingredients—like refined sugars, salt, and MSG—as well as chemicals to artificially enhance flavor, color, and preservation.

Though they may seem harmless, these practices decrease nutrient content and are designed to induce cravings and increase consumption. They have a massive cost to us, and not just in the form of expanded waistlines. Over time, consumption of these foods can have a devastating effect on us internally—on our health and vitality (from lack of nutrients in depleted food) and on our self-confidence (from overeating and giving into cravings). What's happening *inside* our bodies can indeed determine how we feel about our *outside* appearance.

Our biochemistry cannot be ignored.

The quality of nutrients in the foods, as well as their bio-availability, have so much more of an impact on our appetite, cravings, and energy than the quantity, or calories/energy, of the food does. **Bio-availability** is the ability for the nutrients in foods to be digested, absorbed, and used efficiently. The quality and bio-availability of nutrients also affect cell reproduction, which affects *everything*—and for a Forever Body, this is especially vital to know for reducing the effects of aging and for developing lean muscle mass.

If you still think that "a calorie is just a calorie," then changing this belief may be the first place to start. I hope I can help you to shift this belief by sharing with you how I *never* count calories anymore or even look at the "nutrition label" on food; I only read ingredients. And as long as my shelves and fridge are stocked with quality food, I never need to worry about cravings or overeating. This, I believe, is one of the (many) underlying principles behind my Personal French Paradox experience, too: the French are known for their quality food.

Choosing more whole, natural foods instead of processed, refined ones is, hands down, the #1 habit that's helped me to feel fantastic about and in my body every day. In fact, I probably eat *even more* food now than I used to when I "counted" everything. But, because it's full of nutrients that my body can digest and use more efficiently, I never feel heavy, sluggish, or bloated—and I haven't had to buy bigger clothes in a *very* long time.

The great thing is that there are now more companies catering to health-conscious consumers. This means that, from time to time, I can still buy a bag of potato chips or cookies, ones that are actually made with ingredients I'd use myself if I'd made them by hand. So I'm not deprived at all, and this is a *big* key to maintaining results over the longer term.

Yes, these novelty health foods can sometimes be a little costlier. But since they don't make up a large percentage of my shopping items, it doesn't bother me to splurge on the occasional sweet or savory treat that I don't have to make myself. (I also happen to be a nutritionist who doesn't like to spend hours on end in the kitchen when I could be out doing other things!)

When we consider that *everything* we eat needs to be processed through our bodies, and that the food (chemicals and all) we ingest can indeed alter our physiology, it's a small price to pay for higher-quality products and ingredients that provide—instead of deplete—important nutrients for our optimal functioning.

Food quality is the key.

The bottom line is this: through modern food processing and manufacturing practices, our food has become so low in nutrition that, no matter how much of it we eat, we can still be starving.[24] Our bodies will continue to crave more food until they get the nutrients they need to function optimally—and because they generally don't get enough, they're always wanting more.

This is especially critical to note with "portion-controlled" foods; they are usually purely calorie- or fat-focused, not nutrition-focused. So, while you may be keeping your caloric consumption low, or within "weight-loss range," your body will be in constant craving or starvation mode because it hasn't been nourished enough. This makes it extremely difficult to maintain a low-calorie plan for any extended period of time.

But there's more than just nutrient starvation going on under the surface. Processed and refined food can induce other physiological effects, which I believe are truly stronger than our willpower could ever be. These are inflammation, impaired digestion, and blood sugar imbalances.

I'll go into each of these in a little more detail.

Inflammation

Inflammation is how our bodies react to, and protect and heal us from, potentially harmful pathogens or injuries. But it can also be a response to the food we eat.[25] If our food is loaded with toxic chemicals (additives), and/or with ingredients that we're not capable of digesting efficiently (as is the case with most processed food), it can indeed create an inflammatory response in our bodies in the form of general swelling, puffiness, and bloating.

Our bodies are very smart and they will do whatever they possibly can to keep us in a balanced state. When our bodies are so focused on protecting us, they will hold onto the inflammation for dear life until it's no longer required (that is, until we stop putting stress on our bodies—physically and emotionally).

Even if we don't have a detectable food allergy, our bodies can still have a sensitivity to certain foods.[26] Many ingredients in processed/refined foods can trigger inflammation, and anyone who consumes them regularly could be carrying around an extra 5 to 25 pounds of excess water weight.[27]

Rapid weight loss at the beginning of a diet can often be attributed to loss of this water weight. When we reduce the amount of food we eat, this can help reduce our inflammation. This is a good thing, but simply reducing food intake alone won't provide long-term relief. Calorie-reduced diets aren't easily sustainable, and one day of "cheating" can quickly pack the inflammation weight right back on. A better approach is to improve the quality of the food we eat, so that food-related inflammation eventually becomes a thing of the past.

Holding onto inflammation weight can be very discouraging, especially if we're religiously following diet guidelines and seeing little to no result. If you're following a diet which also includes packaged/calorie-controlled foods and you're feeling discouraged—not to mention hangry (hungry plus angry)—this could be why.

It's worth noting that *stress* can also be a huge source of inflammation. When we aren't getting enough of the appropriate nutrients (due to nutrient-deficient food intake... do you see the common theme here?) that our bodies need to fight stress, this can compound our inflammatory response. So, aside from reducing or eliminating refined and processed foods, managing our stress also becomes a critical factor in helping to minimize inflammation.

Impaired Digestion

This particular physiological response is one that I feel extremely passionate about because the dieting stress that I put on my body for years seemed to have the most profound (negative) impact on my digestive system. I battled IBS for several years until I studied nutrition and learned to heal this over time. Irritable Bowel Syndrome (IBS) is a term used to describe digestive distress for which a structural diagnosis can't be made—it's more of a "functional" disorder, usually characterized by chronic gas, bloating, constipation, and/or diarrhea. (It's not to be confused with the more serious Inflammatory Bowel Disease (IBD), which includes Crohn's disease and ulcerative colitis.)

I remember getting so frustrated with the pain and discomfort I would experience every time I would try to eat "better": diet-approved meals, calorie-portioned snack foods, basically everything that was labeled "100 calories," "low fat," "high fiber," or "gluten-free."

It was only when I started learning about and reading ingredients—and making decisions based on the *quality* of the foods, rather than their claims—that I began to feel more comfortable physically and more confident in my ability to choose supportive foods more often. And when my gut healed, my cravings decreased.

• •

BUYER BEWARE: So-called health claims on product packages are usually there for marketing, not health, reasons. Smart marketers quickly catch on to trends. Now that I'm more aware, I laugh each time I see a gluten-free label on something that never contained gluten in the first place, like a bag of potatoes or coffee. Same goes for a cholesterol-free label on vegetables (as cholesterol is only found in animal products). But I actually get angry when these labels are on packaged foods full of artificial ingredients and chemicals—especially on products aimed at children. This is why it's so important to educate ourselves and not rely on package claims alone.

My digestive tract is now a well-functioning machine most days, and it's quick to tell me when I've eaten food that doesn't support it, so I can confidently say that improving my digestion was the best motivation to help me develop and maintain a healthier relationship with food.

What I learned is that the chemically altered ingredients in processed foods put an enormous amount of strain on our digestive systems. The result? A seriously uncomfortable and harmful combination of *nutrient depletion* and *toxic overload*.

Malnutrition can result from weakened digestion and absorption, and it's a risk that we all face. We are indeed a society that is overfed and undernourished. I truly believe that the biggest reason we eat more than we need to is that we didn't get the nourishment our bodies needed from our last meal. Our bodies are still starving for life-sustaining micronutrients and will often respond with more hunger and cravings. Even though the stomach may be physically full, the body's cells are still starving!

Not only are these foods nutrient-deficient (stripped of nutrients in their processing), but they also cause us to tap into our bodies' own storage of minerals to help digest them, which depletes us further. We need minerals to digest our food—something that nature provides for us so well in natural, unprocessed foods; therefore, once our stores are depleted, our digestion suffers even more, which causes more indigestion, gas, bloating, and constipation.

As a result, we're loaded with even more toxins to deal with: those from the ingredients themselves and those created by our bodies as a by-product of the impaired digestive process. The removal of fiber in the processing of food doesn't help, either. Without it, there's essentially nothing to help move things along through our systems, which further compounds the toxicity problem.

To illustrate how this resulting toxicity and malnutrition can thwart our efforts for achieving a lean, healthy body, here are a couple more specifics:

Stubborn Fat

What's one of the many negative effects in our bodies when we have an increase of toxins in our system? Stubborn fat. Since our fat cells are part of our bodies' protective mechanism, they're a great place for us to store toxins so that they won't cause extra stress on our organs. The more toxins we have in our bodies, the more we need to hold onto that fat.

Our abdominal area gets most affected by this; it's where visceral fat literally packs up around our vital organs for protection. Potentially leading to cardiovascular disease, among other health concerns, this kind of fat is the most dangerous kind (as opposed to fat on our hips and butt), and it's also the most difficult to lose.

If you've ever had the experience of losing weight but not fat, especially around the belly, toxic overload could be part of the reason. It's *not* just about the calories.

Heavy Gut

(Warning: poop talk coming up!)

Did you know that you could be holding up to ten pounds (or more!) of compacted waste in your colon? If you're not eliminating regularly (often a result of consuming low-fiber, processed foods), you could be hauling around extra weight, which can be naturally remedied with some simple digestive support.

It's normal to be carrying around a few pounds of poop—as the colon is a constantly working machine that's not meant to be totally empty. But constipation can often be the cause of unnecessary discomfort and distress (both physically and emotionally), as well as unwanted "heavy" belly weight.

When my daughter, Eve, was younger, she would often hilariously state, "Mommy, pooping is the best part of my day!" And I have to say, after overcoming years of chronic constipation, I can totally relate to that statement! Can you? If you're not regularly having great-day-making poops, this may be an aspect of your health worth examining a bit closer.

How do you know if you're "regular"? Well, each person's body functions differently so there's no single right answer, but, ideally, food transit time (from ingestion to elimination) will be anywhere from 24 to 30 hours [28]—which translates roughly to one poop a day. According to some schools of thought, we should even have three poops a day (one for every meal). But my belief is that one good poop per day is enough for most people to maintain great health. Any less than that, and we're probably getting into the category of "heavy," unnecessary belly weight.

To clarify, the nutritionist's definition of a "good poop" is one that is

- effortless (no strain),
- mild in odor (someone could walk in after you and not hold their breath),
- not too hard, too soft/loose, too light, or too heavy (the "Goldilocks" poop has the consistency of toothpaste and drops gracefully to the bottom of the toilet),
- brown in color (unless of course you've had some beets),

- about the length of a large banana (a whole banana, not a chopped-up one), and
- making you feel like a million bucks (like you can relate to Eve's comment)!

If you're not currently having at least one of these a day, every day, then this problem could be partly to blame for excess weight or feelings of heaviness, particularly around the waistline. The good news is that, with a bit of time and commitment, it is entirely possible to get things working regularly and efficiently and to make every day a great day. Isn't that exciting?

> Great poops can lead to a great life! In other words, improve your digestion and you improve your destiny!

As a nutritionist, I'm pretty passionate about poop talk (if you haven't noticed). It's such a central component of overall health—and of your Forever Body—that if it makes you at all uncomfortable reading or talking about it, I lovingly encourage you to get over it. All weight-loss discussion aside, the reality is that constipation can lead to serious illness if not resolved. And illness is definitely not supportive to living out your greatness or even living happily, for that matter.

In short, great poops can lead to a great life! Or, in other words, improve your digestion and you improve your destiny! (I'm only sort of kidding.) Okay, moving on from poop ...

Here are some tips that may help you to start improving your digestion:

- Chew your food thoroughly; digestion starts in the mouth.
- Eat more raw foods; they still have their natural enzymes and nutrients intact.

- Drink more water; staying hydrated helps prevent constipation (drink away from meals, so you don't dilute digestive juices).
- Eat more mindfully; avoid eating when distracted, upset, or stressed.
- Take digestive enzyme supplements with meals (to assist immediate digestion and to reduce gas and bloating).
- Supplement your diet with probiotics; more good bacteria equals more good poops (and they also boost the immune system!).
- Eat more sprouts and naturally fermented foods (for example, miso, kefir, and sauerkraut), as these are natural food sources of enzymes and probiotics.
- Increase your fiber intake; flax and chia seeds are a couple of my faves (wheat bran is generally a poor choice as it can be too harsh and may cause more harm than good).
- Choose whole, natural, and minimally processed foods more often; this is the way nature intended for us to eat them.

And, for extra poop support, exercise daily, get proper sleep, and poop in a "squatting" position (since modern toilets aren't designed to accommodate our natural pooping position, you can create this same effect by propping your feet up on a step stool).

You may also wish to seek the support of a qualified naturopath or nutritionist who can help you to navigate through your personal digestive situation, if it's a particular concern for you.

Blood Sugar Imbalances

. . . .

If you've ever experienced an energy "crash" after a sweets binge "high," you're probably familiar with the effects of a blood sugar imbalance. You can usually recognize low blood sugar by its symptoms of dizziness, headaches, anxiety, irritability, excessive sweating, and/or lack of focus or concentration—followed by ravenous hunger and sugar cravings to relieve these symptoms. If you know what I'm talking about, I probably don't have to tell you that this physiological response easily overpowers your willpower—you've felt it for yourself.

Here's a simplified nutritional breakdown to illustrate what's happening in our bodies when we eat sweets (carbohydrates)—and how processed, refined foods can wreak havoc on our blood sugar balance and therefore our willpower:

When we eat something sweet
or starchy (in normal quantities):

Carbohydrates (sugars and starches) go into the digestive system and are broken down into their components—glucose, fructose, and galactose—which are then absorbed into the bloodstream.

Our blood transports these to our liver, where everything gets converted to glucose—*the body's main fuel for energy*. The liver decides how much glucose stays in circulation (blood) for immediate energy and how much gets stored for later use—in the form of glycogen, for short-term storage, and fat, for long-term storage. (Note: the only way that sugar gets converted into fat is when there is too much of it in our system for immediate or short-term use. See the example in the next section.)

The glucose remaining in the blood gets carried into our cells as needed, by the hormone insulin (created by our ever-helpful pancreas). The cells' mitochondria then produce our energy, and all is well. (Did I mention this was a simplified explanation?)

This process is slower for complex carbohydrates (starches) than for simple sugars, as it takes longer to digest and break them down into glucose. However, both are good sources of energy.

When we eat too much of something sweet (like in processed, refined foods):

Carbohydrates go into the digestive system and are *quickly* broken down and converted into glucose. Too quickly.

Too much glucose ends up in the bloodstream (creating a temporary sugar high); and in its efforts to balance the blood sugar and restore homeostasis, the pancreas produces *too much* insulin to help carry the glucose *too quickly* from the bloodstream into the cells where our mitochondria use it to produce energy.

But since there's *way more* glucose than we need for immediate or short-term energy, the excess gets promptly converted to fat. (Fat is simply the best "just in case" storage system. It's very efficient at holding onto our potential energy for very long periods of time. So if we ever find ourselves in a state of famine, our fat stores will be there for us!)

In the meantime, back in the bloodstream, there is a homeostatic emergency: the blood sugar has become too low (aka hypoglycemia). The *excess insulin* production caused *too much* of the sugar to be transported out of the blood at once, and now we are in a state of low blood sugar.

So, what's the best way to bring the blood sugar back into balance? You got it: more sugar—and fast! This state can lead to overeating, usually of the wrong things. Often it involves eating anything in sight to get relief of these symptoms quickly.

The problem really escalates when we do this all day, whether we know it's occurring or not. If we are eating packaged, processed, and refined foods regularly, we could be experiencing this up-and-down cycle multiple times a day. Even if we're not eating "sweets," *refined* complex carbohydrates in our everyday foods have a very similar effect to sugar, as they are quickly broken down into glucose. Therefore, foods and ingredients like white flour, white rice, and anything made with them (pasta, bread, couscous, cookies, muffins, bars, cakes—you name it) are also dangerous contributors to our blood sugar imbalances—even if they are "calorie-reduced."

By eating calorie-reduced processed foods that contain *refined* carbohydrates, we can actually make it harder on ourselves to reduce our consumption of sugar.

Fat-reduced products can also make it worse. For starters, "low fat" foods are typically higher in sugar, because sugar is frequently used as a flavor compensator in the absence of fat. Also, since fats—especially the healthy kind—can help to slow down our digestion and uptake of glucose, the absence of fat in these products contributes even more to the problem of blood sugar imbalances.

But "carbs" aren't necessarily the enemy!

Sugar, and "carbs" in general, are currently a hot topic among dieters. They've been given a bad name, and, in many ways, this reputation is warranted. Refined sugars and starches, present in so many of our packaged and prepared foods, are undeniably at the root of our obesity and diabetes epidemics because they're overconsumed.

But carbohydrates are actually vital nutrients to our optimal functioning, for the following reasons:

- They're our main source of energy (for body and brain).
- They're needed to digest and metabolize protein and fat.
- Our immune system would be faulty without them.

We'd also be missing out on our main source of fiber without complex carbohydrates—something we absolutely want to avoid, as I mentioned in the previous section on digestion.

From a "balancing" perspective, carbohydrates also help to reduce our cortisol levels (the "stress hormone") and carry serotonin (our "happy hormone," also a natural appetite suppressant) into the brain. This may explain why, during times of stress, many people crave and turn to their favorite carbs for comfort, not necessarily out of hunger (and why it's also important to address stress in the big picture, too).

Therefore, carbs are *not* the evil enemy. The real problem with them lies in *the quality and quantity* in which they're currently being consumed in the Standard North American Diet. Sugar is in literally every processed food (read the ingredients!), and it's the most refined it could possibly be. This can make it very difficult for us to

> Carbs are *not* the evil enemy. The real problem with them lies in *the quality and quantity* in which they're currently being consumed in the Standard North American Diet.

succeed at limiting our consumption, no matter how committed we are.

What makes me sad, though, is that the pleasure of eating sweets and starchy foods is being stripped from us by the toxic processing of our food. Let's face it, life without *some* carbs is really no fun at all—they can add so much pleasure to our eating experience, if consumed moderately. Seriously, how many Atkins dieters are still out there? Who wants to live without the pleasure of sweets forever?

Since carbs have become "bad" or "forbidden" foods (as confirmed by numerous popular books and diets), these classifications are making an increasing number of people feel guilty when they do consume them. Because avoiding carbs is not natural, or easy to do, this can lead people further down the low-self-esteem rabbit hole.

I strongly believe that *everyone* deserves to enjoy comforting starchy dishes, delicious baked goods, and chocolate on occasion—even every day if they choose—and to not feel guilty about it or have it negatively impact their health or weight. (This is why quality is key!) I'm therefore here to help you embrace a new relationship with "sweets"; give up the fear of carbs; and return to enjoying them regularly and moderately, in their whole, natural form.

An important note on artificial sweeteners

Despite our best intentions, the use of artificial sweeteners as substitutes for sugar can actually have a negative effect on weight-loss efforts (and on our health, but that's another story!). The most commonly used artificial sweeteners include aspartame, acesulfame potassium, saccharin (Sweet'N Low), and sucralose (Splenda).

Contrary to popular belief (which marketers are incredibly skilled at engraining in us), these artificial sweeteners do not help you lose weight. In fact, research has shown that consuming artificial sweeteners can actually increase appetite and cravings for carbs, and promote weight gain.[29]

The simple explanation for this is that they confuse the body's metabolism. The body receives something sweet (which appeals to the immediate pleasure/sensory reward), but it doesn't get the expected accompanying calories for energy. Therefore, it continues to crave more sugar and carbohydrates for the missing energy, which then leads to increased appetite.

So, next time you're adding artificial sweetener to your coffee or tea, or choosing "sugar-free" options from the bakery or candy store, I urge you to think twice. There's a multitude of natural alternatives that will not harm your health or cause weight gain, if consumed in moderate amounts, and they still taste delicious.

Here are some tips for satisfying your sweet tooth on a regular basis, without guilt, and without consequence:

- When you eat something sweet, include a source of fiber, protein, or healthy fat to decrease the transit time of glucose into the bloodstream (keeping blood sugar more stable).

- Enjoy *moderate* amounts of less-processed, nutrient-rich, and more satisfying sweeteners, such as unpasteurized honey, pure maple syrup (not table syrup), coconut palm sugar, blackstrap molasses (not "Fancy" or "Cooking" molasses), and raw cane sugar. Just keep in mind that natural sugars can still cause imbalances. Options that have little to no effect on blood sugar balance and are still satisfying to the sweet tooth, include Xylitol (a sugar alcohol that also benefits dental health) and Stevia (a naturally sweet plant).

- Bake your own sweet treats with quality, whole, natural ingredients—or find a healthy, reputable bakery that does the same.

- Choose chocolate containing *at least* 65 to 70% cocoa, as darker chocolate is typically lower in sugar and higher in health benefits (especially if you choose organic). You may have to retrain your palate to appreciate the flavor, but it's so worth it!

- Eat a variety of fruit—either by itself or combined or blended with a handful of nuts, seeds, coconut chips, organic cheese, or yogurt.

Know that there are plenty of ways to get your sweet fix without harmfully disrupting your blood sugar levels or your health and weight. You can use these tips, as well as the resources provided at www.FindingYourForever Body.com/Resources as a great starting point.

I assure you, it *is* possible to shift your relationship with sweets, carbs, and food in general. I've done it, and I hope to help you do it, too, so that you can feel that you're nourishing and satisfying your mind, body, *and* soul on a daily basis. This requires making choices that serve *all three*, and that's why a "diet" just won't cut it for the long term.

2

A Unique Solution

· · · · ·

Changing for Good

. . . . .

WHEN I LOOK back at my journey, I can see clearly that it was not an overnight process. And I'm still evolving. Every year on my birthday, I still feel like I can see improvements in my health and fitness (and as a result, in my life, too!) from the previous year.

But any permanent result I've had did *not* come from a diet—and I'm positive that anyone who's ever had success at *maintaining* a healthy weight over the long term would confirm that this has also been their experience. For the record, I'm not referring to the "naturally skinny" type who can eat anything and never put on weight. I've often been identified as belonging to this category of people, but, trust me, if I suddenly became sedentary and wasn't mindful of my habits, it would be clear how wrong this classification is. I'm talking about the average person who maintains a healthy body weight and size, and who doesn't do it through dieting *at all*.

I've learned that people who have maintained permanent change over the long term, without dieting, have done something very simple that sets them apart from those who are stuck on the vicious diet cycle: *they've developed and maintained supportive habits.*

They know that there is no perfect diet plan, and they've given up the fruitless search. Instead, they've adopted habits that they know will support them over the long term, while letting go of the need for short-term, quick fixes. They acknowledge that they're on a journey and that they're building on their results over time. They also take pleasure in the fact that, while they're doing this, they can get on with their life right away...

Sounds very simple, but it's not easy for most people. And that's because there's a foundation missing: *core self-esteem.*

I firmly believe that most people know intuitively what their bodies need to feel good, and *the reason they don't do what supports them has very little to do with lack of knowledge.* Most people know that fresh, whole, natural foods are good for you and that refined, processed foods are not. Most people know that physical activity leads to good health, and being sedentary does not. But if everyone followed the basic guidelines for good health, we wouldn't have the overweight and obesity rates that we currently do, and the diet industry wouldn't be the giant that it is.

Self-esteem and supportive habits work hand in hand to get us where we want to go. When our self-esteem is high, it's easier to keep up our supportive habits, and when we keep up our supportive habits, we feel better about ourselves and our self-esteem is higher.

But there are so many distractions in our environments that can pull our focus away from who we are and what we want to accomplish. No one is immune to this, and we can easily become disconnected from ourselves if we don't have the proper structures in place to build and maintain our strong foundation of self-esteem.

I developed the ten steps in this section based on my own experience of what helped me to lift my core self-esteem, develop my own intuitive self-care daily practices (aka supportive habits), and maintain them for good, no matter what is going on in my life.

These are strategies designed to help you successfully break up with diets and the scale once and for all, to nourish your body with ease, and to fall in love with your body in the process.

Now, let's begin . . .

*"I've been on a diet for two weeks
and all I've lost is two weeks."*

TOTIE FIELDS

Step One:
Ditch the Scale

· · · · ·

I REALIZE THAT this may contradict every piece of weight-loss advice you've ever heard, but that's why this book is different. There's a very good reason that I've made this the first step: I believe that it's the most important step for laying the foundation for a new way of being with your body.

So, I repeat, please, *ditch the scale*. The number that it shows you is only a very small indicator of your overall health, and it probably makes you feel bad about yourself more days than it makes you feel good. I know this from experience. Get rid of it.

The scale gives you a number. That is all. It doesn't measure your inner beauty, your strengths, your gifts, or your worth. Yet so many of us have been sold on the idea that the number is the ultimate goal, that if and when we achieve our "goal" weight, then we'll feel worthy, accepted, and happy.

You see, we've been sold on the idea that our self-worth can be measured by a number (on the scale, tape measure, or dress tag). No, the ads don't word it that way, but that's the underlying message. We've bought into a set of standards that have been established by outside sources, and the metrics are all wrong.

Looking back, I see the irony in the fact that I wanted to become a model in the ads that encourage these unrealistic standards, and yet I didn't meet them! (I only saw the blessing in this *many* years later...)

To give you further insight into just how messed up the standards are, I'll share with you a bit more of my experience meeting with the "big time" modeling agency when I was 17.

After showing up excitedly for my much-anticipated go-see, I confidently sat down opposite the agent and handed her my comp card (a printed headshot photo, with height, weight, and other measurements on the back). Here's what it read:

Kim
Age: 17
Eyes: Blue
Hair: Blond
Height: 5′8½″
Weight: 137lbs
Chest: 32″
Waist: 28″
Hips: 36″

> The scale gives you a number. That's all. It doesn't measure your inner beauty, your strengths, your gifts, or your worth.

She examined the card, then me, and said: *Well, you're a little too short for us to take you on. We require our models to be at least 5′9″. You're only 17, though, so there could still be time to grow.*

You're also too heavy. Sometimes, we can overlook the missing height—as you're only half an inch too short, we might be able to consider you if you met our weight requirements. At your height, you should weigh no more than 125 pounds.

Come back when you've lost the weight and grown a bit taller, and we'll see if we can reconsider you then.

As if that wasn't earth-shattering enough, she added:

Oh, and your crooked bottom teeth should be fixed if you want to succeed in modeling. I'd look into getting braces, too.

Even though I quit modeling after that, I'd already bought into the idea that I wasn't good enough at 137 pounds and had unacceptable "imperfections."

I also continued to allow external sources to dictate my self-worth. I weighed myself daily. In my younger years, my body was fairly forgiving of my binges and I could lose a few pounds quite easily after packing them on. I always managed to keep my weight within a range of 135 to 140 pounds, sometimes getting down a few pounds lower when I was feeling "mentally stronger."

Even though I'd enjoyed freedom from the scale during my stay in France, I became even more obsessed with it than ever afterward, especially as I felt my weight go up. During my post-France/pre-nutritionist years, my weight hovered in the 145-to-148-pound range, and I was weighing myself *up to six or more times a day.*

I remember weighing myself first thing in the morning, after breakfast, before and after lunch, before dinner, and before bed—and if I ever had an opportunity to use someone else's scale for comparison's sake, I would. I'm not even kidding. If I was your dinner guest and you had a bathroom scale, I would use it, both before *and* after dinner. It was a big problem.

I never felt good—physically or emotionally. The first time I started feeling any freedom from the stress I constantly placed on myself was when I decided to put the scale away for good. I finally decided that measuring myself by these metrics was fruitless and I had to find another way to feel good about myself and my efforts.

These days, I typically step on a scale about once a year and, according to the scale, I'm heavier now at 41 years old than I was at 17, as most people tend to be. But I'm also now the most fit I've ever been in my life, and I feel completely confident in my body—which was never the case when I was scale-obsessed, even when I'd reached my lowest weight.

If I had allowed the scale to continue to dictate my self-worth all these years, I can assure you that I'd be no further ahead in my journey. I'd be stuck. Stuck obsessing. Stuck dieting. Stuck on the daily roller coaster of moods that fluctuated with the number on the scale.

Scale obsessing is indeed one of the most unsupportive habits facing most people who struggle with their weight and body image. For me, even though I *knew* that achieving a weight of 125 pounds was nearly impossible to do without starving myself, I continued to strive for the impossible—while watching the scale go in the opposite direction, as I

· ·

As sick as this may sound, during my diet-cycle days, I sometimes even found myself *envying* people who suffered from anorexia, because I thought they had more willpower than I could ever have. Since I had developed a fear of starving from my earlier dieting experiences, I couldn't commit to such severe food restriction, and I attributed my failure to achieve my goal weight to this mental "limitation."

continued the pattern of restricting and bingeing. Even after returning from France and modifying my goal to 130 pounds (still ridiculously underweight for a healthy body of my height) to try to set myself up for "success" finally, I still felt like a failure, because I was never able to achieve it again. As you can imagine, that didn't help my self-esteem much.

It wasn't until I started my studies in holistic nutrition that I started to understand what I was really committed to, what really motivated me. I realized that what I truly wanted was to *feel* good—and to *be* happy! And the scale couldn't measure those results for me.

My weight was just shy of 150 pounds when I began my studies, and I'd almost given up on the possibility of getting anywhere near 130 pounds—though it was still in the back of my mind as my "ideal weight." Thankfully, by this time, reaching the number on the scale had become secondary to feeling good—after years of dealing with poor digestion, a compromised immune system, and low levels of energy and concentration, all caused by dieting.

It's amazing what happened when I started to focus on the quality of food I was eating (to feel good), rather than on the calories (to lose weight). Not only did I find it much easier to commit to *adding* in health-supportive foods, instead of restricting my food intake, I also found that I could better understand my body's cues for hunger and satiety, and avoid the pattern of restricting and overeating. I lost a bit of weight over time, but, more important, my body started feeling and looking healthier than it ever had in my entire life—and the number on the scale became much less of a consideration.

Today, the scale is now a totally obsolete tool to me. And I hope to help you make it obsolete in your life, as well. In order for you to begin to put a stop to the vicious diet cycle and the emotional toll it can have on your self-esteem, the scale must go.

I actually hope that, one day, scales will be banned everywhere but in doctors' offices. Why not just leave it to the doctor to measure your weight as *one* component (of many) of your overall health—and *only* if your weight is a health concern? If it's not in the overweight or obesity range, there are much better ways to track success toward a healthier body and lifestyle.

So how *can* you measure your success? How will you *know* if your efforts are paying off and you're heading in the right direction?

We'll get to that soon, I promise (that's a Step Three question!). But, first, it's time to start separating your size, weight, and shape from your self-worth.

Step One Actions Checklist

- ☐ Locate your bathroom scale.
- ☐ Get rid of it (hide it, trash it, donate it . . . make it disappear!).
- ☐ Resist the temptation to use someone else's scale.
- ☐ Forget about the number (the "goal weight").

"To be yourself in a world that is constantly trying to make you something else is the greatest accomplishment."
RALPH WALDO EMERSON

Step Two:
Love What You've Got!

. . . . .

Starting with the Inside...

THERE'S MORE to lifting our self-esteem than feeling good about our bodies. More important, we need to feel good about *who* we are.

Do you know the answers to the following questions? If not, I encourage you to spend as much time as you need in this step—before proceeding any further—to get really clear about your value and worth, particularly to yourself:

- What are your strengths?
- What are your gifts, passions, and talents?
- What do you love about yourself?
- What do your friends and family appreciate about you?
- What makes you feel alive?
- What contributions do you make to your community?

This is the stuff that really matters. *This* is your real beauty. However, what tends to happen—for women, especially—is that we get so distracted by our efforts to meet external standards regarding size and "beauty," that we forget to focus on the *real value* that we have to offer. For a moment, let's shift the focus completely away from your physical appearance, and take a deeper look within.

We all have our own *unique* internal qualities, and we can't discover them by looking around us. It's a self-exploration process. Unfortunately, we live in a perfection-obsessed society, where we're constantly looking around us to see how we measure up. (How many self-proclaimed "perfectionists" do you know? I'd guess it's a lot.)

Perfectionism isn't limited to our image or appearance, either; if we develop this habit in one area, it easily transfers into others. Think about how many times you've put yourself down for being "less than" what you see around you—for some reason or other. I know, for some it's a scary thought; from my own experience, I can't even count that high!

But we can't all be great at everything (that would be exhausting), and perfection is, in fact, a completely unrealistic and paralyzing goal. If we feel we can't do something "perfectly," it may stop us from doing it at all.

In this step, the pursuit of perfection is being replaced by the pursuit of authenticity: discovering what makes you you *and then unapologetically allowing those qualities to shine.*

Have you ever wondered how seemingly beautiful, slim women could feel insecure about their bodies? (I've learned that models are, in fact, some of the most insecure people on the planet.) Or why celebrities, who were never overweight to begin with, develop eating disorders?

It's because so much of their value has been tied to their external appearance, to their overall image—and this puts so much undue pressure and focus on *shit that doesn't really matter* in the grand scheme of things! Not only is having a "perfect" image unimportant in the big picture, but it will always be impossible to measure up to society's standards of "perfection." They are not realistic, and they never take into account the beauty in our individuality—in our uniqueness.

Our image is *not* who we are. I learned this the hard way…

I struggled so much with my body image growing up because I had put so much of my energy into an extra-curricular activity that focused exclusively on my image: modeling. I placed way too much value on my appearance, and I measured my success and worth by it, which inevitably transferred to other areas of my life. And then, after all I'd put into it, I was rejected for not being enough. My image wasn't enough, and therefore I felt that I wasn't enough; I felt I had failed because I didn't measure up.

Only after a long journey of discovering more about *who* I am and identifying the metrics by which I can truly measure my success, did I begin to develop the self-esteem to sustain supportive habits and to be happy with my body and my life in the process.

So, here's my request: instead of looking around you to identify your standards and success markers, and then beating yourself up for what you are *not*, try this much more empowering approach:

Begin to look within to highlight and build on both the positive qualities that you possess and what you have to offer the world. (I personally believe that everyone's here for a reason.)

Recognize that you can be loved and appreciated *for* your "imperfections" because they make you human and they are part of *who you are.*

The more you can embrace yourself, from the core to the surface, the more you can feel free to be unapologetically, authentically *you* and to start living your life as you want to live it *now.* This self-acceptance will no doubt lead you to develop and sustain habits that support your healthiest, most vibrant physical body yet.

Here's why this inside-out approach works: when we start to focus on the gifts we do have, rather than what we don't have (perfect body, skin, etc.), we can truly begin to honor our bodies as the vehicles that support us in physically carrying out what we're really here to do. And when we keep an eye on the bigger picture, measuring ourselves by external standards eventually becomes a thing of the past.

We can start taking care of our bodies because we honor them for their role in transporting us through this life. We can begin to nurture and nourish them in the best way possible so that we have the energy to pursue the passions, and care for the people, that matter to us.

We are given only one body in this lifetime to carry us through to the end, and we're blessed if we have all our fingers and toes and our mobility. Yet most of us go through life punishing, depriving, and abusing our precious bodies in an attempt to fix them like they're broken. But unless we stop breathing, they're never really broken.

Our mindsets are, though. Marketers have broken us by selling us on a damaging set of standards, tricking us into believing that achieving them will help us to love our bodies. But it's all backward. We have to love our bodies—and, more important, ourselves—first.

When you take the time to do this work—and truly get to the heart of what your *strengths* are—you are, in fact, laying a stronger foundation on which to achieve and maintain your physical goals (weight loss or otherwise). There are two main reasons why this work is imperative for your Forever Body:

1. It helps you establish your sense of self-worth: your value to yourself. You'll start to believe that you *deserve* to live in a healthy, vibrant body for the rest of your life. If your mind isn't set to focus on developing and strengthening your own self-worth first, no matter how much you transform your physical body, your results will be short-lived. Your mind will always match your body and vice versa. So if you maintain a low sense of self-worth (thinking that transforming your physical body alone will lift it), your long-term habits will reflect this, and eventually your physical body will return to a state that reflects this, as well. But if you begin to transform your mindset as you set about achieving your physical goals, your long-term habits will support your increased sense of self-worth, and your body will indeed cooperate.

2. It leads you on the path that's best suited for *you*. When you get really clear about the qualities that you value in yourself, you can better choose which programs, products, activities, behaviors, and habits will be best suited for *you*. They'll be the ones that intuitively speak to you— and you won't buy into everything that's being sold to you. This will not only save you a ton of money, but it will also help to accelerate your progress toward your goals.

And Let's Not Forget about the Outside!

Identifying and building on your internal strengths is the first, and most significant, aspect of loving what you've got, but this step also involves loving what you see when you look in the mirror, right now. This is one of the hardest things to do, which is why it's critical to start looking at yourself as a *whole* being—who has an inside and an outside!

With the knowledge of your inside strengths and beauty, you'll find it easier to give yourself permission to love and accept your outside—pimples, dimples, and all! This means being able to face the mirror directly, look at all aspects of your body, and appreciate the entire vessel for what it does for you—for how it allows you to be here and to live this life now. *All* parts of our bodies have a function. They weren't just created for show! Once we're able to look beyond appearances, we can start to pour love and gratitude into each and every nook and cranny of our physical bodies.

> Know your inside strengths and beauty, and give yourself permission to love and accept your outside—pimples, dimples, and all!

Moving away from judgment and toward gratitude is simply the process of really getting to know your entire physical body, without relying on any outside measurements. (If you've completed Step One, it should be easier to resist weighing yourself!) It's also the means by which you can start to nourish your body, because our actions are a reflection of our thoughts. When we turn our thoughts to the positives—to gratitude—our actions follow suit; and nourishment, not punishment, becomes our path to long-term results.

To illustrate what I'm saying, imagine if someone you loved, in an effort to change or improve you, tried to do so through means of punishment, deprivation, or, worse, by withholding love. How would you respond? Chances are, you might make changes in the short term to appease this person, but eventually you would likely rebel or retaliate. Our bodies are no different. They respond to love and nurturing much better than they do to actions driven by negativity.

Body love must come first, before any long-term change can be sustained; and to love and accept your body, you need to get to know it! Here's an exercise to help you do this:

1. Stand naked in front of the mirror. No matter how uncomfortable this makes you feel, knowing how you look naked is fundamental to your self-awareness. When we're ashamed of our physical appearance, we tend to hide it. But if we want to develop true self-acceptance, we need to come out of hiding. So get comfortable with your naked self!

2. As you stand there, you will no doubt immediately want to point out the things you dislike, but it's important to do this without judgment. When you notice areas that you want to improve, stop and switch your thoughts immediately to finding something that you can love about them right *now*, before you even change a thing. (For example, if you notice saggy boobs, acknowledge and love them for their role in nourishing your children.)

3. Be sure to also acknowledge and pour gratitude into those areas that you *already* love, or even like, about your physical self. (We all tend to have at least one or two of

these.) Maybe your eyes? Your smile? Your complexion? Your sexy hourglass shape?

4. Next, notice what makes your physical appearance unique—what makes your body special and different from any other. Celebrate your differences; you weren't made to be like anyone else, inside or out.

If you find this to be a difficult step for you (our minds can be great saboteurs when they want to be), I've also created a *Self-Talk Detox* guided body-love meditation to help you subconsciously replace negative thoughts about your body with new, more empowering ones. You can access it for free at www.FindingYourForeverBody.com/Resources.

Step Two Actions Checklist

☐ Answer these questions to acknowledge your inner beauty:
  · What are my strengths?
  · What are my gifts and talents?
  · What are my passions?
  · What makes me feel alive?
  · What do my friends and family appreciate about me?
  · What contributions do I make to my community?

☐ Stand naked in front of the mirror and acknowledge what you love about your body, and give gratitude for your unique traits. For "areas of improvement," find something to love about them before you change a thing. (Ask yourself, what does this part of my body do for me? What has it done for me that has added value to my life?) If you are living and breathing, there is always something positive to acknowledge.

☐ For help with this process and to eliminate negative self-talk about your body, download the *Self-Talk Detox* guided body-love meditation here: www.FindingYourForeverBody.com/ Resources.

"The starting point of all achievement is desire."

NAPOLEON HILL

Step Three:
Feel Your *Real* Desired Outcome

. . . . .

MANY PEOPLE HAVE health goals like "I want to lose xx pounds" or "I want to get down to x percent body fat." But, as I mentioned earlier, I believe that their "magical willpower" is often absent from their quests to achieve these goals because they fail to get to the root of *what* it is that they really want and *why* they want it.

In other words, until you identify your *real* desired outcome, it will be nearly impossible to solidify your commitment to maintain your willpower over the long term.

It's worth repeating that *everyone* has willpower; what is actually lacking, in most cases, is real commitment. Now, before you object to this statement, I want to first clarify the difference between wanting something and being committed to it.

Wanting something may be prompted by many different things: societal pressure, envy, or even the belief that achieving it will somehow make your life better. *Being committed* comes from solidifying *why* you really want it; and this has to start with identifying what *you* really want—and why *you* really want it. Nothing and no one else can determine this for you; it needs to come from *you* and resonate with *you* to your core: emotionally, physically, and spiritually. When you truly get in touch with *your why*, you'll be instantly blessed with magical willpower! It's really quite astounding.

From this point forward, I encourage you to always replace the word "willpower" with "commitment," which will help you to examine your goal more closely to see if it's something you even want and, if so, to ask yourself *why*. This step encourages you to examine your motivation with a fine-tooth comb.

Before we get further into this chapter, I'd like to point out a truth that may surprise you: weight loss (that is, achieving a number on the scale) is probably not what you *really* want. How do I know this? It's a bold, generalizing statement, but I truly do believe it's the case for most of us.

I'd like to show you how I've reached this conclusion by sharing more details about my own turning point (for the better), when I'd reached a state of depression.

Emotionally, I was feeling completely trapped in my life. My body seemed like the enemy—an annoying distraction that kept me from being able to make healthy changes in my life because I couldn't stop obsessing over its imperfections.

Physically, I also was unwell—a side effect of the diet cycle, which had me constantly gassy, bloated, and uncomfortable after eating. I was completely exhausted most mornings, even when I slept in. And I was sick *all* the time: colds, bronchial infections—and even at one point, an undiagnosable illness that covered me head to toe in an itchy rash, with so much inflammation that you could hardly see my earrings! If you had asked me then how I felt most days, my honest answer would have been "like a bag of crap," though I hardly ever answered honestly.

My stress, combined with less-than-ideal nutrition, had zapped all my energy and vitality. But I knew I couldn't settle for a life of depression and sickness, and I finally reached a point where I realized that, without my physical health and energy, it would be impossible to move forward with the changes I wanted to make.

I knew I had to make peace with my enemy.

Earlier in my life, I wanted to change my body *first* and feel accepted and worthy *first* so that I could move forward. This time, however, being miserable helped me to see two things:

1. I needed to move forward with my life *now*.
2. My body was going to be the supportive vehicle that would transport me through the important changes I wanted to make.

I had always known that I had internal gifts and strengths that had been ignored in favor of my body-image obsession. But, at this point in my life, the pain of not honoring my true spirit was finally greater than the pain of being heavier than my "ideal" weight.

My body transformed from my enemy into my best friend and ally. And my health goals changed, too:

I no longer wanted to lose weight; I just desperately wanted to feel better and more energetic.

I wanted to improve my digestion so that I could feel comfortable after eating and throughout the day.

I wanted to heal my relationship with food so that I could spend my energy on more important things than counting calories and measuring portions.

I wanted to relearn to eat intuitively, like I'd done as a kid, so that eating could become a natural and pleasurable (not forced or controlled) experience again.

I wanted more ease, flow, and balance in my life—and to feel the sense of freedom that I knew was possible.

But I couldn't see any of these goals materializing if I kept going in the direction I was headed. And even though I had these health goals, they weren't really my motivation for changing my behaviors and habits.

My *real* motivation came from envisioning *the life I really wanted* (my why).

Interestingly, the next focused steps that I took in my life had nothing to do with my body, and yet, with each step I took, my body did indeed change—as nutrition, fitness, and good mental, emotional, and spiritual health became foundational elements for helping me move forward. Here are the first pivotal self-discovery and life-changing steps I took:

1. I left a depressing corporate marketing job to pursue full-time nutrition studies.
2. I left my unfulfilling marriage and home with little more than my car, my shoes, my books, and my cat.
3. I moved across the country (to the west coast of Canada, where my heart had been calling me to go for years) to start my life over again with no idea of the next step . . .

None of this would have been possible without my health. Nor would any step I've taken since, and there've been many to get me where I am today. I'm now in a place where I feel *completely* aligned, and many dreams have become realities (including waking up to watch the sun rise over the ocean and mountains without even stepping out of bed). I assure you, I wouldn't be here if I was still allowing my body image to define my self-worth.

I share this story with you because it wonderfully illustrates the fact that weight loss is never the *real* goal. There is always an underlying, more motivating desire—something bigger than changing our physical appearance. Usually, it's the *feeling* of happiness and self-confidence we *think* we'll achieve when we feel better about our appearance that leads us to focus on changing our bodies first.

But what I've learned is that being happy and confident—and feeling beautiful, for that matter—is an inside job, and it can't be achieved by simply losing weight. However, weight loss and good health *can* result from being happy and confident, which, in turn, comes from pursuing a path that is in alignment with what you truly want for your life.

So, your question for self-reflection is: *What do I really want?*

Be specific. I recommend that you start by making one big list of desires—pertaining to relationships, job, home, city, social life, travel adventures, athletic endeavors, and anything else that comes to mind. I found it particularly helpful to think of and write down my "ideal day." What would your ideal life look like, from the moment you wake till the moment your head hits the pillow at night? Describe it in as much detail as possible, so you can then extract the main themes for change. (That is, what parts of your ideal tomorrow most differ from your today?)

What Do I Mean by "Feel" Your Real Desired Outcome?

It's not only important to identify and "see" what you want; you must also *feel* it. What does this mean? It means *imagining* the outcome, in detail, and really *feeling* what it will be like to achieve your desired changes before you even consider *how* you will get there. (Don't allow the unknown of "how" to distract you from your visualization.) If you are clear about *what* you really want (you can see it), and *why* you want really want it (you can feel it), the *how* (process, steps, programs, opportunities, support, etc.) will reveal itself along the way.

Writing your thoughts out in a journal is a great way to work through and identify *what* you truly want for your life. Once you've got a good laundry list of desires, you can narrow in on *one* that you'd most like to achieve first—the one you can start to work on right away. The good news is that *all* areas of our lives are connected, so improving any area will inevitably cause a positive domino effect on the others.

Once you've chosen that one desire to focus on, you can solidify your *why* (your commitment) by asking yourself the following questions:

- How will it feel when I achieve it?
- How will it change my life, and even my relationships?
- What will I be able to accomplish once I achieve this?
- What will happen if nothing changes?
- How will I feel if I never achieved this?
- Is this goal—and the steps I would need to take to get there—in line with my values? If not, what is? (It's important to be clear on your top values.)

What Does This Have to Do with Your Forever Body?

. . . .

Here's what makes this process completely different from any other weight-loss or body-transformation approach: by *first* getting clear on what you want for your life, and why you really want it (a solid commitment), you can then ask yourself:

What support do I need from my body in order to achieve this "ideal" life?

This will then serve as your foundation for setting your health goals—and I'd be willing to bet the answer doesn't come just in the form of a number on the scale. Describe the ideal state of health that will allow you to pursue your ideal life.

It's crucial that you take the time to do this exercise *before* setting out to accomplish another health or weight-loss goal, because there will be times when you will want to give up, and that is when you will look to *why* you wanted this goal in the first place. (Most people's diets and fitness regimens peter out by February because they're missing this foundation.)

In my case, my biggest desire was to run my own business, work from home, and help people with their health and nutrition, from anywhere in the world. I value freedom and fulfillment, and was feeling neither through my corporate job or lifestyle. But my body definitely wasn't in a good enough state of health for me to pursue leaving my job and starting up a business—and I also wasn't walking the talk of a health practitioner. So, I set some health and fitness goals to increase my energy and vitality so that I could pursue my dream.

Are Your Goals SMART?

It's fantastic to have goals, and I believe that it's absolutely essential to set clear ones in order to achieve the things you want in life, including a healthy weight and body.

I've spent most of my adult life setting goals each year, month, and even week. I learned from an early age that it's important to write down goals as part of the process of achieving them. Our chances of accomplishing them significantly increase when we write them down.[30]

What I've found, though, especially in the case of my health and body-weight goals, is that writing them out simply wasn't enough. In fact, I've got years and years' worth of journals, in which the same weight-loss goals are repeated, over and over again.

So if I wrote them down, why was I never able to achieve them? The answer is simple. They weren't SMART.

The SMART acronym has been used for decades as a goal-setting guide in business and personal development. There are some variations to it, but the most widely used version of it stands for

Specific
Measurable
Achievable
Realistic
Time-Bound

But I've modified it here slightly, with our Forever Body in mind, because using some of these guidelines could be problematic if you're committed to breaking the diet cycle. For example, "lose ten pounds in 30 days by eating only

1,000 calories a day" may be specific, measurable, achievable, realistic, and time-bound, but it's not a Forever Body goal. When it comes to improving your health, there's no deadline (unless, of course, there's a medical reason, like impending surgery). Finding your Forever Body is a journey, not a destination.

Instead, Forever Body SMART goals are

Stimulating
Measurable
Attainable
Rewarding
True to *You*

Using my personal experience here as an example, I'm going to walk you through the process of setting and revising your goals in order to set yourself up for successful permanent change.

Stimulating

Does the goal inspire you? Does it make you want to get up in the morning to take the next step toward achieving it?

In my case, simply reaching 125 pounds in order to feel accepted was never a stimulating enough goal for me to follow through on any fitness or diet effort to lose weight. However, the following goals were indeed very stimulating for me:

- increasing my energy naturally (without stimulants),
- improving my mood (without a prescription), and
- healing my gut so I could feel comfortable after eating, rather than gassy and bloated.

These goals are what motivated me to study holistic nutrition, which led to even more positive change than I had even imagined.

At the risk of sounding like a broken record, I encourage you to look beyond the number on the scale—and to think long term. Losing ten pounds in 30 days may be a good goal in your mind, but what happens after 30 days? What would you need to do or give up to be able to lose the weight so quickly? What would reaching your goal weight actually do for you 30 days from now?

I mistakenly thought that reaching my goal weight would allow me to stop obsessing over diets and the scale, and move on to focus on better, more important things. I thought I needed to first lose the weight before I could tackle the next goal, professional or otherwise. I didn't think I could have the focus and confidence I needed for my other goals until I achieved the "acceptable" weight of 125 pounds.

What I failed to realize at the time was that I didn't find reaching my goal weight stimulating enough because I knew it would involve deprivation in order to achieve it (and I wasn't excited about this).

But when I eventually set the goal to improve my energy, I was way more motivated. My energy level had become a big problem, since my low-calorie (and low-nutrient) food choices depleted me on a daily basis. Despite my generous caffeine consumption, I still reached for midafternoon pick-me-up sweets and beverages; I still crashed by the end of my workday with little energy for exercise; and I still could never make it through a movie or evening show without falling asleep on the couch.

I would have rated my energy level *very low*—especially for my age—and I was desperately envious of people who had naturally high energy levels. (Granted, I met very few of these people in my daily life—but when I did, they left an impression!) Improving my energy, so that I could pursue my dream of becoming a health professional and successful entrepreneur, became a very stimulating goal for me.

So, what's a stimulating health goal for *you*? I invite you to now eliminate any scale-related goal that you may have set for yourself before, and set some new health goals that relate to the *feelings* you desire. Also, identify how achieving them will help you work toward your bigger desires for your life.

Think of the positive changes to your physical health that would *really* make a difference and accelerate your progress toward your bigger desires.

Perhaps it's improving your energy level, cardiovascular fitness, strength, sleep, focus and concentration, sense of calm, ability to deal with stress, digestion (lack of gassyness, bloating, and constipation), mood (positivity, fun, and laughter), how you feel first thing in the morning (aka your morning-ness), how rested you feel after waking, how sexy you feel, how comfortable you feel in your clothes, how you feel naked … These are simply some suggestions. I encourage you to brainstorm your own—based on your big *why*. *You* will know best what resonates with you.

Write out a list of as many things as possible that you'd like to see improve in your health, or your relationship with food or your body, and then narrow it down to the *one* that would have the greatest impact on all areas of your life if it were to change for the better. Start with that one as your first goal to work toward.

Measurable

How will you know when you've achieved, or even progressed toward, your goal? This is why it's important to set a goal that you can measure—something other than the number on the scale. (Has this point sunk in yet??) There are more important metrics you can track.

Fitness goals are generally pretty simple to track: gyms and personal trainers usually have metrics to measure your improvement in strength, endurance, and flexibility over time. But other health goals may be a lot more subjective, so it's important to get to know your body and how it feels.

I'm a big fan of the 1-to-10 scale, where a 1 rating is poor and 10 is ideal. Take inventory of your starting point: Where are you now? You want to have a way to measure your progress. You may even want to note in your journal some feelings that describe your current state in more detail.

My personal goal of naturally increasing my energy (without caffeine or stimulants) was measured using a scale of 1 to 10, and I kept a daily journal as I made changes, in which I recorded my progress, along with other life events. When I started, I rated my energy level at a 3 to 4. Now, I rate it at 8 to 10 most days. There is also a stark positive difference in the quality of my life today compared to when I began my journey, which is no coincidence.

Aside from a journal for capturing your thoughts and progress, another great tool to use is a daily *Food, Fitness, and Sleep Tracker*. (I've created a downloadable PDF template for you, which you can access here: www.Finding YourForeverBody.com/Resources.) But this is *not* for recording calories. This tool is simply for recording each day how your body responds to:

- food (what you eat and how much),
- fitness activities (what, when, how much, and how intense), and
- sleep (when and how much).

As you make changes, you'll likely see your body's responses changing, too. Using this measurement tool may take a little more work in the beginning, but gaining these insights is an immense help for getting to know your body and what adjustments you may need to make along the way.

As you'll see in the tracker template I've provided, you can also record your energy level, mood, and digestion using a 1-to-10 scale, as they can be greatly impacted by food, sleep, and fitness. (And feel free to also track other metrics you've identified for yourself.)

WHAT ABOUT TRACKING WEIGHT-LOSS RESULTS?

I can't pass through this "measurable" section and totally ignore the fact that many people like being able to see the tangible *physical* results of their efforts. If I'm encouraging you to ditch the scale (and the tape measure), then how can you measure your progress if your goal is to lean out your body?

Here's one technique that I feel is much more intuitive (aka in tune with your body) than relying on measurement tools like the scale, tape measure, or fat calipers: use what I like to call your "benchmark pants."

Most of us have a pair of pants (or shorts) that we can use as a benchmark to measure our current size. They must be pants that do not stretch after wearing or shrink in the wash and they must represent a healthy size for you (not necessarily your "skinny" pants—I'm talking about your long-term, sustainable, feel-good-size pants).

Try them on now and note (on paper—even in your journal) how they feel, where they're tight, and whether or not you can do them up! This will serve as your beginning measurement. (You can even take a picture of yourself in them to help you remember your starting point.) Then pack them away for a month or two before trying them on again. Do not try them on every day or even every week. Your changes will be slow and steady, and therefore your progress will be, too.

Attainable

Is your goal realistically attainable? Maybe you have a goal, like I did, to reach a weight or size that doesn't seem feasible

• •

IMPORTANT NOTE ON "BEFORE" PHOTOS

I'm also a proponent of taking "before" photos because they can provide you with a sense of accomplishment by allowing you to visually see how far you've come toward your goals. However, I don't recommend displaying them where you can see them every day. (If you see yourself in a "negative" light, this is not a great source of motivation.) So if you do take "before" photos, simply file them away—they will be great to dig out later on when you're celebrating your success.

Be sure to take photos not only of your body but of your face, too. Internal improvements to your health and happiness can definitely be seen and "measured" through changes in your skin, eyes, and hair.

without drastic measures (that is, you've tried everything but starving yourself, and nothing has worked). If you do, then it's time to trash that goal altogether—because it's only setting you up for failure. (I hope you've let go of your weight-loss goals by now.)

Or perhaps your bigger goal *is* attainable and realistic, but it seems like you have such a long way to go that it feels daunting. In this case, it could be helpful to break down your giant, lofty goal (which is still good to keep in mind) into smaller, measurable, more attainable mini goals, or sub-goals.

For example, getting to an 8-to-10 energy level right now may seem totally unrealistic given where you're starting from, so you could break that down into smaller steps, like first reaching a 5 or 6. Or if you want to run a marathon, but you're currently out of breath running from the car to the house, then you may want to start by setting a 5K goal, and build up from there. Or if you're a night owl who stays up till 1 a.m., but you want to start going to sleep by 10 p.m. to improve your productivity and energy, then you may set an immediate goal to go to bed an hour earlier. Once you've nailed that, set your goal for another hour earlier. You get the point . . .

The best way to make your bigger goals attainable is to break them down into manageable sub-goals. Taking away the overwhelm, and adding in feelings of accomplishment, helps to more quickly build momentum and keep it going.

Rewarding

What forms of gratification will you get from achieving your goal? When we set Forever Body SMART goals, we don't need to reward ourselves for the accomplishment because our reward can come from the achievement of the goal itself. What do I mean by this?

By increasing my energy level to an 8, 9, or 10, I have the energy to do so many more things in my life: stay active with my busy daughter, take on new fitness challenges, build a business that I love, embark on new adventures, write this book! I also feel as though I'm walking my talk as a health coach and nutritionist. (Who would want to work with a health coach who's exhausted all the time?) And I'm attracting wonderful people into both my life and business, which is a beautiful reward.

I also love a challenge, so when I had the goal to improve my energy, I took it on as a "mission" to complete. I experimented with food, sleep, and supplements until I found the formula that worked for me.

What do you find rewarding? Do you like the sense of fulfillment that comes with learning? A challenge? Competition? Recognition?[31] As you're setting your goal, it's important to be clear on the rewards you'll get, both by achieving *and by pursuing* it.

True to *You*

Is this goal really *yours*? Make sure that you're reaching for these goals for *you*, not for anyone else. And not to be accepted or respected by your spouse, friends, coworkers, or, in my case way back when, the modeling industry. Your goals must be *true to you* in order to fulfill *all* the rest of the SMART criteria.

When I look back at my weight-loss goal, it's clear that it wasn't established by me. It was set *for* me by a modeling agent. I had allowed someone else to place in my head the number I needed to achieve. My goal wasn't even mine!

Now when I set new goals, I always use this experience to remind myself why it's so important to ensure that they are in fact true to *me*.

Step Three Actions Checklist

- ☐ Identify what you *really* want for your life—make a list and choose one desire to focus on.
- ☐ Solidify your commitment (your *why*): what will it really feel like to achieve this desired outcome? Use the questions on page 96 to help you.
- ☐ Ask yourself: What support do I need from my body in order to achieve this?
- ☐ Make a list of as many things as possible that you'd like to see improve in your health, or your relationship with food or your body.
- ☐ Choose the one that would have the greatest impact on all areas of your life if it were to change for the better.
- ☐ Set SMART goals to help your body achieve that supportive state of health. Start with one.

> *"Do not wait to strike till the*
> *iron is hot; but make it hot by striking."*
> WILLIAM BUTLER YEATS

Step Four:
Start *Now*

· · · · ·

CHANGE STARTS with a decision, not a date.

If you're committed to changing your health and lifestyle in any way (if you're still reading, I'm guessing you are), start now. Take *one* step toward it today, and, before you go to sleep tonight, you will have come one step closer to your goal. Isn't that exciting?

The problem with the way most people approach change, especially when it comes to changes in their body, is that they wait for the "perfect" start date—after they've completely planned and prepared for the drastic changes they are about to make. This puts so much unnecessary pressure on themselves and on the date, and it's a "short-term result" mentality.

The only way to sustain changes over the *long term*, and maintain *permanent* results, is to start *now* and start *small*. And plan and prepare as you go—this is a journey after all!

This is not just a suggestion; it's an essential step to prove to yourself that you're serious about change. Don't wait. There will never be a more perfect time to start than right *now*. I don't care if it's a Friday or December 24—here's the most important distinction between dieting and living healthy and well: realize that *any day* is a good day to start living the rest of your life the way you want to live it.

I can't stress enough how important this step is.

So, what's the best way to start now? Start small. I mean, ridiculously small. *So* small in fact that if you told someone what your action step was today, they might think (or even say), "What's the point?" That reaction just highlights the problem with the way things are currently done, with the quick-fix mentality, and with diets in general: we've been programmed to make drastic changes and expect fast results—and to have to restart over and over again.

> The only way to sustain changes over the *long term*, and maintain *permanent* results, is to start *now* and start *small*.

This is exactly why the diet industry is thriving and we are not.

Your Forever Body does not come from a quick fix. It comes from regular, consistent action that develops new and more health-supportive habits—over time. That may not be the answer you were hoping to find in this book, but it is truly the only way to achieve *permanent* results.

Think about this for a moment: How long have you had your weight-loss goal? Be honest with yourself. For me, it was almost 15 years that I was striving for the magic number I thought would bring me happiness. If someone had told me upfront that following these steps would help me reach a state where I would *never again* have to set a weight-loss goal—even if it took five years to get to that state—I would have gotten here much sooner. Ten years sooner, in fact. And truthfully, it didn't even take five years once I discovered this baby-step approach as a key to changing for good.

This slow and steady approach generally isn't the most popular one because it doesn't usually bring drastic visual results in a short time frame. But, as they say, "slow and steady wins the race." And small, incremental changes *do* bring big results—because when changes are small and manageable, and they don't turn your life upside down overnight, they're much easier to sustain for the long term. Imagine, if you start this today—making a commitment to one small change daily—by this time next year, you will have made 365 permanent changes.

This strategy compounds results, builds momentum (and confidence!), and definitely pays off in the long run. Even if you only made one change per week, you'd still have made 52 permanent changes in one year! Isn't that way better than ten drastic, unsustainable ones that you have to repeat each and every January?

The vicious diet cycle of starting and quitting over and over and over again, which has plagued millions of people, is holding us back from living truly fulfilling lives. It held me back—big time. My weight, and my apparent failure to achieve the desired number on the scale, was a huge distraction that kept me focused far too much on my body, instead of the more rewarding and fulfilling projects and life goals I wanted to work toward.

Every time I tried something new, I expected fast results (so I could finally move on from this distraction as quickly as possible). But I would easily grow tired of that effort when it didn't give me the results, especially if that was a promise of the product or program. Then I would move on to find the next best thing that might.

What I didn't realize at the time was that each time I embarked on a new diet or eating plan, I was setting myself up for failure. Why? Because I was making too many big changes at once—giving up foods and habits, trying to embrace new ones. I was also giving up a lot of my life (time and other priorities) to incorporate these changes, which wasn't sustainable at all. Inevitably, I would give up when it got to be too hard, frustrating, limiting, or, worse, boring.

In time, and through my studies of nutrition and my curiosity about habit formation, I developed a new philosophy that has worked very well for me over the years: each change I decide to make needs to be something I can continue forever (unless, of course, I find that it really doesn't give me any joy).

Before I start anything new—take any new step—I ask myself: *Is this step something I can imagine doing for the rest of my life (if I choose to)?*

If the answer is no, I make the change smaller until the answer is yes.

I urge you to do the same: *only* take on changes that you can reasonably sustain forever—which means they will sometimes have to be ridiculously small. That's not to say that you won't *eventually* get to bigger, more impactful steps, but in order to take consistent, daily action, your changes need to be doable and sustainable for two reasons:

1. To give you an energizing and motivating feeling of accomplishment when you complete them (versus the

feeling of failure you get when you set your expectations of yourself too high and can't follow through).

2. To build your momentum (before you know it, you'll be doing things that you may never have thought possible ten years ago).

Taking the First Step

The first step is often considered the hardest—which is why we usually put off starting until Monday. I'm not sure if this belief has contributed to the diet mentality, or if the diet mentality has created this belief. No matter which came first, this belief is *not* supportive of permanent change.

Here's a new, more empowering belief: the first step is always the easiest.

It should be setting us up for success! That very first baby step should be something that we can easily check off our to-do list, laying a piece of the foundation, so that we can add one more tomorrow.

So how do we choose our first and subsequent baby steps? Well, let's remember again the meaning of the word "diet": it simply refers to the food you eat, to what you put in your mouth. And I'm assuming that you put food in your mouth every single day (or at least you should). So, today, make one thing you put in your mouth a little better for you than what you ate yesterday—even if it's just one meal or one item. Then make one more change tomorrow and another the day after that. Keep going. That's how small steps eventually begin to compound into bigger results.

The following considerations may also serve as a guide for determining your small, manageable, daily actions:

1. Always focus on the positive.

Adding things to your diet and lifestyle is usually a much more sustainable and enjoyable approach to change than *taking things away*. For now, focus on steps like adding in foods that are supportive to your health, energy, digestion, etc., rather than on eliminating foods that you're meant to avoid. (You'll probably find yourself naturally gravitating toward elimination eventually.)

Substitutions are another positive approach so you don't feel like you're completely missing out. Replace something you know isn't serving you in achieving your goals with a similar-tasting, more health-supportive option. I've listed some of my favorite substitutions in my online *Nutrition Resource* (www.FindingYourForeverBody.com/ Resources).

To stay focused on the positive, it's important to remind yourself regularly of *why* you want to achieve your health goal in the first place (see Step Three). From that starting point, you can more easily switch your mindset from one of deprivation ("I can't eat that. I'm on a diet.") to one of nourishment ("I'm going to ensure I eat an energizing superfood smoothie for breakfast so that I have the energy to do X today.").

2. Recognize that it's okay to "try on" a variety of approaches—that's part of the self-discovery process!

Developing your own supportive diet and lifestyle is like putting together the perfect wardrobe for you. You'll need to shop around, try on many things, see what fits, and buy *only* what makes you feel your best. Keep what works and dismiss the rest.

What looks great on your best friend may not suit you quite as well, and vice versa. Our outsides are designed differently, and so are our insides, right down to our cellular building blocks. It's imperative to remember this, and to enjoy the shopping process—it's half the fun! And if you hate shopping, let your "personal shoppers" help: that's what professionals like nutritionists, personal trainers, and coaches are for. You never have to shop alone.

3. Start by narrowing in on *one* habit that you want to change at a time.

Commit to changing that one habit first, before you even look at other areas of your life. By putting all your focus on that one area, you'll increase your chances of successfully changing that one habit; and more often than not, changing one habit, especially in the area of health, will have a domino effect on other areas of your health and your life. All areas of our lives are connected; none exist in a vacuum.

4. Remember that *quality > quantity* when it comes to achieving your Forever Body.

This equation applies both to food and to fitness, and the first step to applying it is to begin learning what quality really is: start educating yourself, find reputable resources (don't just rely on marketing and package claims), and, most important, learn to listen to and trust your body.

Granted, there's so much to learn, and it can all seem quite overwhelming. That's why it's crucial to remember that developing a healthier, leaner body is a *process*. Although it won't happen overnight, every better food and lifestyle choice does make a difference. If you think of the fact that our bodies are made up of trillions of cells that are reproducing *every second*, and that the nutrients we absorb from our food each day form the building blocks of every single one of these cells, you can start to see the bigger picture. What we eat doesn't just determine how much we weigh; it also determines how well our cells, organs, and systems function. This obviously has an enormous impact on our overall physical, mental, and emotional well-being.

APPLYING THIS EQUATION TO YOUR FOOD

Opt for choices that nourish you, satisfy you, and give you sustained energy. When you do this, and when you obey your body's natural hunger and satiety cues (more on this later in Step Seven: Do Your Hunger Homework), you won't have to worry about counting calories—or fat grams, or carbs—at all. As I mentioned earlier, it's much more important to focus on where your food is coming from, how it's produced, and what ingredients it contains.

I also encourage you to stop buying into the myth that you can eat everything in moderation; otherwise you could end up eating your entire day's worth of energy (calories) in moderate amounts of crap food—and starve your body of critical nutrients in the process. Even if the calories are low enough to allow you to lose weight in the short term, the weight loss won't be sustainable because your body will be starving.

APPLYING THIS EQUATION TO YOUR FITNESS

Don't underestimate the power of 30 minutes a day. You don't need an hour or more to get your fitness on and get results! There are plenty of effective, high-quality workouts that you can get done in a short amount of time—which will also help to increase your chances of successfully making fitness a regular habit.

Getting a quality workout also means doing something that you enjoy. If it's not fun, it's not likely to stick over the long run.

5. Take pleasure in the process— and acknowledge your progress!

Permanent, positive diet and lifestyle changes are driven by a positive shift in our overall outlook on life, which is a result of being happy *right now*. In other words, each of us is on our own journey, even though it may not be "perfect"—and we're meant to enjoy this life *now*. Not just later on, when we achieve our goal. Now. When you set yourself up for success by setting Forever Body SMART goals and taking baby steps, and you acknowledge and reward yourself for your *progress* along the way, you will be able to have a much more enjoyable journey.

> Don't wait until you get to your destination— celebrate your milestones, too!

One Step at a Time—Literally

I'm going to share with you a story from my personal life, where this baby-step approach really stood out as a key tool. I feel that this example in particular is a great metaphor for any desired change or goal...

One day when I was 24 (and still living with body-image struggles), I was driving with my then-boyfriend, and we stopped briefly at a store to pick something up.

It was raining, and so I lightly "jogged" from my car into the store to avoid getting soaked. When I returned, he was laughing at me:

"I can tell you're not an athlete," he said. "The way you run—ha!"

Well, that relationship didn't last, but I can tell you that his comment stuck with me for a long time afterward. I'd always secretly dreamed of running a marathon, thinking that would be a hell of an accomplishment to aim for in life. But he was right: I had never been an athlete and it was obvious. I decided that I wanted to change that, and so, fueled by a desire to prove whoever wanted to judge my apparent lack of athleticism wrong, I started on the journey to make that change.

I decided that *learning to run* would be a great start. One might think that running is just something we should all be able to do naturally because our bodies are designed to do it—just the same way we're designed naturally to eat. However, in running—just as in eating—there are ways to increase our pleasure and decrease our chance of injury (or illness), so it's great to be able to benefit from the experience and expertise of others.

The first step I took was research. I learned that proper footwear is important for running.

The next step I took was going to a running store to ask the experts' opinion on shoes, and I bought a proper pair.

Then I joined a "learn to run" clinic.

Then I started to run. My first run consisted of five one-minute running intervals, with two-minute walking breaks in between—my initial workouts totaled no more than 15 minutes.

Then I decided I wanted a challenge and I signed up for a 5K race.

Then I found a training program. For months, I ran three to four times a week, gradually increasing my running times each week until I was running for ten-minute intervals with a one-minute break in between.

When the week of my race arrived, I was feeling strong and confident, and I decided last minute to change my registration for the 10K instead. Race day, I ran my heart out and completed it in under an hour (a time I was very proud of for my first race), but I was in pain afterward. I had caused injury.

I waited for my injury to heal, and then I started over. I had to go back a few steps but not entirely back to the beginning.

I discovered a true love of running and have been running ever since (on and off, having to recover from various injuries—'tis the life of an "athlete," I've realized!). I haven't done a lot of races in that time, but I've maintained running as a part of my fitness regime because I enjoy it immensely.

When I turned 38 (14 years after I started running and feeling happy in my body), I decided it was time to challenge myself again. I registered and trained for a half marathon, and completed it in under two hours—again, a finish time that I was very proud of but which, again, caused injury.

It took me almost 18 months to heal that injury and get back up to running distance. But, after having to stop and heal and refine my stride, posture, and even shoes to prevent injuring myself further, I realized that I was finally ready to run my first marathon. I'd collected all the tools and confidence I needed; all that was left to do was train for it.

And I did it. I trained for and ran my first marathon last year, to celebrate turning 40.

I tell you this story to illustrate how big results come from regular small steps over time—not from giant leaps overnight. They require commitment and consistency, not groundbreaking technology.

I went from being a *very obvious* non-athlete to a marathoner who can't imagine life without running—and who now even enjoys other athletic endeavors, too. It took 16 years, and it all started with the first step. Followed by another. And then another. Even though I've had to take some steps back a few times, these apparent obstacles or delays ultimately helped me to become a healthier, stronger runner by showing me areas where I still needed to improve. Nothing points out a weakness better than an injury!

If I had started out with the intention of running a marathon as my first race and followed a marathoner's training schedule right out of the gate, chances are very good that I would have either injured myself quite quickly or been discouraged by my lack of cardiovascular endurance and inability to complete a training run without feeling like my lungs would burst.

For me to feel like a marathon was actually within my grasp, I needed to build up my physical strength and

. . . .

Many people get discouraged and feel bad about themselves when they take steps back. But I urge you to start seeing the blessings in setbacks. There's always something to learn that can give you an advantage with moving forward; if you can find and apply the lessons in each obstacle, you can use these to eventually take bigger steps forward. I would even say it's important to take steps back in your long-term health journey. I call it the *Forever Body Dance!*

endurance; my knowledge and self-awareness; and my confidence. And all those components came to me over time with small, manageable steps.

So, here's the key: begin to incorporate changes *now* (like, today) that are sustainable and that you can see yourself maintaining and building on for the rest of your life. This means starting small—sometimes ridiculously so—and knowing that even making one small positive change is a step in the right direction.

Running Your Own Race, at Your Own Pace

Think of achieving your personal desires (from Step Three) as running your own marathon. (Nope, I'm not yet finished with the running analogy. Even if you have no interest in running, please stay with me here—it's a crucial point to be aware of if you truly want to break free from dieting for good.)

For a *very small* percentage of the population, running a marathon is a manageable and regular feat. But for most of us, it's a huge undertaking, and it takes a lot of commitment and effort to even reach the start line.

If you *really want to achieve something*, it's not about how long it takes to get there. It's about staying consistent in your actions and not quitting—and learning and growing along the way. Most people who run marathons are not elite athletes and are not doing it for competition; for most of us, it's about going for a personal best or even just crossing the finish line. I remember reading about a 100-year-old man from India who ran the Toronto marathon in 2011. He finished in just over eight hours! A good story to remember if you ever think "it's too late" or "I'm too old."

The same philosophy can be applied to all our personal health, weight, and fitness goals. Staying committed to our goals, and taking small steps every day, will give us the fuel to keep going toward that finish line, no matter how long it takes. Delays and obstacles are a natural part of life, and if you've done Step Three thoroughly, you won't let them throw you off track. (They may slow you down, but they won't stop you.) You can be more patient with the process.

Remember, there's *no deadline* when it comes to permanent change and finding your Forever Body. Even if you're preparing for a wedding or another big event, chances are that the people who invited you (or your spouse-to-be, if it's your own wedding) asked you to be there because they love you for who you are, not for the size you are. Just know that if you start small today, by the time of a special occasion or target date, you will have progressed from where you are now.

When we diet, it's like starting off a marathon by sprinting. We can go fast for a short period of time, and we may even gain some momentum and confidence from it, but inevitably we crash before reaching the finish line or end goal. We will most likely end up discouraged, quitting the race entirely, which necessitates reevaluating, finding a new strategy, and trying again next time (this perpetuates the diet cycle).

The New Year's resolution comes to mind as the most popular "marathon" on the planet: it's the start line that millions of people rush to each year, typically at a time when they're the most out of shape, most stressed out, and most run-down. Despite this, they decide to "start a marathon" without training. This not only leaves them unprepared physically, mentally, and emotionally, but it can also cause more damage than they realize—to their self-esteem, self-confidence, and self-belief—when they inevitably "hit the wall" and can't follow through to the finish line.

The "Monday" is another popular race, one that I was personally very familiar with during my diet cycle days. It was only when I started seeing every day as an opportunity to train—not race or sprint—that I really started seeing results.

Something I've learned both through my health journey and through my actual marathon training is that the real change, improvements, and results come from the training, not from simply crossing the finish line. And the training is nothing but a self-improvement strategy to start building your belief, your self-awareness, and your will to follow through. Training for a marathon isn't just about running; it's also about shifting your mindset, so that you can confidently show up at the start line, *believing* that you can cross the finish line. And that's exactly the mindset we need for achieving our Forever Body for good.

Step Four Actions Checklist

- ☐ Choose *one* (small) thing you can do today that takes you *one* step forward.
- ☐ Ask yourself: *Is this step I'm about to take something I can imagine doing for the rest of my life (if I choose to)?*
- ☐ If no—make the step smaller until it's a *yes*.
- ☐ Do it.
- ☐ Repeat daily.

"Confidence is preparation.
Everything else is beyond your control."
RICHARD KLINE

Step Five:
Establish the 4 Ps of Your Desired Lifestyle

· · · · ·

YOU MAY HAVE heard of the 4Ps of marketing before—but these 4Ps are very different! They are extra support tools to help you stay on track once you've solidified your commitment and taken that first step.

Here are the 4Ps of your desired lifestyle:

1. Preparation
2. People
3. Places
4. Passions

Preparation

Yes, for a true Forever Body, preparation happens after you start! In fact, it's happening all the time and continually evolving with you. With each new milestone you reach, and as you grow into your new lifestyle over time, your preparation tools will naturally need to adjust to support you in your next phase.

Preparation involves a few different elements: visualizing, planning, and preparing your environment.

Visualizing

Although having the feeling and image in your mind of your true desires is a great start, the way to keep them alive and fresh is to have a tangible, visual reminder that you can see every day. There may be times when you will struggle to continue on your path—let's face it, we all have bad days—so it's during these times that you will look to whatever can keep you motivated. But this visual will not only act as a reminder; it will also help you to build your belief that you can achieve it and to attract things into your life that will help you get there.

> What better way to focus on something continually than to have it stare you in the face day in and day out?

Earlier, I mentioned the Law of Attraction (and the RAS)—the idea that what you focus on expands. Having a visual reminder is a way to use that law, to work with the subconscious mind in a positive way. What better way to focus on something continually than to have it stare you in the face day in and day out?

A great way to make this visual reminder is to create a vision (or dream) board and place it somewhere you can easily see it every day. You can put together a beautifully inspiring collage of pictures, quotes, and words that remind you of your desired outcome.

If that sounds like too much work, you can make it even simpler: you can start with a few inspiring quotes on Post-it notes around the house or pictures on your fridge or screen saver. Whatever you choose to do, the important thing is that they're positioned where you will see them multiple times a day and that they're motivating for you.

What do I mean by "motivating"? I mean don't post a picture of an airbrushed bikini model with "perfect" curves. By already determining *what* you really want and *why* you really want it, you will have identified both your bigger-picture desires and your SMART goals, so ensure that your vision board aligns with these.

And *have fun* creating this visual tool! Carve out some time (alone or with friends—vision-board parties can be a lot of fun), grab a pile of old or new magazines, photos, or printouts, and start making your collage. Remember, you can always add to it, so don't worry about making it perfect—and definitely don't make it more complicated than it needs to be. It's an ever-evolving project. You will know that you've got a good vision board when it makes you smile and gets you excited to move forward.

Planning

It's essential that you write down and schedule your baby steps every single day, or it's highly likely that they won't get accomplished—especially over the long run. What gets planned and tracked gets done.

Personal planning is a big part of preparing yourself for success, but unfortunately it's often overlooked. And though it may seem like an easy step for those who already consider themselves planners, I'm requesting that you take it even further—I'll explain in a moment. For starters, here are the basics to becoming an effective planner:

1. Keep an agenda book.
2. Use it.

A wall calendar is not enough. Although it's nice to look at and great for keeping track of birthdays and holidays, it's relatively useless as a tool for planning personal success. So if you don't currently have a proper planner or agenda book (with a least two pages dedicated to each week), I urge you to make this your baby step today: go out and splurge the $10 to $20 to get one. If you already have one that's been gathering dust somewhere or feeling neglected, dig it out and crack it open.

Electronic calendars can work okay, too—if you're familiar with and accustomed to using them—but they're not my favorite method of planning. In my experience, there's a much higher chance I'll follow through on activities when I've handwritten them. There's good reason for this: when we write things out by hand, we're registering them in our

· ·

NOTE (IF USING PAPER): Don't use the excuse that there's not much time left of this year so you want to wait and just start with a fresh agenda book next year. *Do not wait*—this is a crucial step to your preparation for long-term success. You may even get a great discount on this year's book. Buy both—the first will be your practice one, so don't be picky. The one that you'll use for an entire year should be one that you will enjoy opening and using often. In other words, choose a design that really represents who you are and what you are out to achieve.

subconscious minds. So, we're in fact giving ourselves an advantage when we write out our baby steps into our paper agenda books.

Now, do you have your agenda book? If yes, please read on. If not, go get one. Seriously.

Okay, whether you're a self-described planner or not, you should now have an agenda book in hand. Next is the tricky part—start using it!

Begin by writing things in your weekly schedule that you already carve out time to do. (This is just practice.) Things like work, kids' events, social activities, phone calls, cleaning, bill paying, doctor's appointments, etc. Just get in the habit of using it. This will accomplish a couple of things:

1. You will get used to using it as an everyday tool for overall effectiveness—in your whole life, not just your goal-driven activities. (It significantly decreases the chances of forgetting things!)
2. You will start to get a sense of how much time you have in a day and how it's divided (especially if you get in the bonus habit of color-coding. I buy a pack of highlighters and have a color for each category of commitment).

Are you spending a lot of time serving other peoples' needs, leaving little time for your own? It's important to account for how and where you spend your time, in order to begin scheduling time to take action toward your goals.

As you get rolling with your baby steps each day, you may need to start shifting things around and reprioritizing. Start by identifying the things you currently do that are flexible and those that are not. Are there things that could either be reduced or eliminated from your schedule? For example, did you say yes when you wanted to say no to a commitment?

Do you need to ask for help, delegate, or even outsource some tasks to make more time for yourself? This will also help you to set clear boundaries around your time and to ensure that you and others respect them.

Beginning to make changes to your health will require making changes to your life and, hence, your schedule. Your agenda book will become your life and health planner—and as you start including your health-supportive baby steps, you can start to treat them like you would any other non-negotiable appointment.

Remember the idea behind the baby-step approach in this exercise. In other words, don't get carried away scheduling "gym time" five days a week, if you're currently getting none. Always take into account where you're starting from, and build up very slowly from there. Scheduling a 15-minute walk, and actually doing it, will make you feel much better about yourself than scheduling an hour at the gym and canceling. You are now setting yourself on a path to make *permanent* changes. Always keep this in mind.

Preparing Your Environment

TOOLS AND NECESSITIES

What physical tools do you need to follow through on your baby steps? Once you identify which steps you will be starting with, you need to ensure you're properly equipped. There are often some must-haves that you need to even get started.

For example, if you want to start swimming or doing Aquafit classes, a good sport swimsuit (that keeps everything securely in!) is important.

Making sure that you have healthy ingredients on hand is also a big necessity for most people. Maybe you also need workout gear (proper shoes, bras, socks, clothes), cooking and baking equipment, recipe subscriptions or cookbooks, or a gym or yoga membership.

When you're equipped and prepared, it's much harder to find excuses for not following through. So make a list of your necessities, and start by acquiring those things that you absolutely can't do without, knowing that you can always add the nice-to-haves as you go.

SAFE AND TASTY SUBSTITUTES

Part of having a Forever Body mentality means knowing which foods you will need to keep out of reach and out of sight in order to avoid going down the rabbit hole of self-sabotage. But it *doesn't* mean avoiding the pleasure that these foods can provide! In most cases, there are wonderful, healthier substitutes that can fulfill the "cravings" without sending you into a tailspin of overindulgence, so it's important to prepare yourself for this properly.

• •

PLEASE NOTE: I'm not referring here to calorie-controlled portions/packages of your favorite refined and processed foods—they can be very deceiving, disguising themselves as "health foods." I once ate an entire bag of 100-calorie chocolate bars (that's like 10 or 12 bars) within 24 hours because I thought they were healthier for me. I would have been way better off just eating one bar of the "real thing," along with an apple and almond butter to balance things out!

With the help of my online *Nutrition Resource* (www.Finding YourForeverBody.com/Resources), you can start to identify which health-supportive and tasty substitutes you may want to store in your fridge and cupboard that will keep you satisfied and on track.

SUPPORT SYSTEMS

Usually, when we think of support, we think of people. But when the going gets tough, it's also crucial to have some of your own systems in place that you can tap into, even when others aren't around. Support is not strictly limited to people, and this is a good thing (which I'll get into in the next P).

The other support systems you can establish for yourself are very much individual—what works for me may not be the best thing for you. But there are several systems you can explore to see what does work best for you. The key thing is that you find something uplifting, motivating, soothing, encouraging—something that can switch you quickly out of a negative state or "funk" when you need it. This may include any of the following systems, and more:

- Having a strong spiritual outlet
- Keeping a journal
- Spending time in nature (the beach is my go-to!)
- Keeping "charts" or logs of your progress, and referring to them often
- Playing your favorite music
- Burning incense or scented candles, or diffusing essential oils
- Reading (or listening to) inspirational and motivational books

One of my favorite ways to get back on track when I'm having a bad day is to head out on a brisk walk. For me, there's something so meditative and healing about the combination of fresh air and low-intensity exercise that allows my mind to clear and my positive energy to return.

Think of what personal strategy has worked for you in the past, or try some new ones, and get really clear on what works for *you*. Be sure to have your personal support systems in place and "at the ready" for whenever you need to access them along your journey.

People

As bad as this may sound, once you begin to improve your health and happiness, not everyone in your life will want to see you succeed—whether they're aware of it or not. Unfortunately, if the people around you feel jealous, envious, or threatened by your success, or if they simply do not understand or relate to your goals, this could sabotage your efforts and impede your progress.

Therefore, it's extremely important to take the time now to carefully consider who you will include in your support network. This means *consciously* choosing who you spend more time with (those who uplift and encourage you), and who you want to avoid (those who drag or push you down, even if unconsciously).

Choose your support network wisely.

How do you choose? Well, the answer to this question depends entirely on your personal situation, but there are some things to consider.

It may seem wise to start by including the people in your home—those in your immediate environment—but this isn't necessarily the case. Although it's a great idea to give them a heads-up that you will be making some changes to your lifestyle, and it's good to ask for their support, don't be surprised if there's some resistance, especially if you've had "failed" attempts in the past. On the other hand, a supportive spouse may be a very good choice if they truly stand behind you in all that you do.

Here are some great questions to consider before approaching a friend or family member for support:

- How has this person supported me through other situations in the past?
- How do I feel about myself when I'm with this person?
- Is this person currently emotionally available to support me?

It's not always easy to find reliable people within your immediate community who will stand by you through the good and bad days on your journey. There may only be one, and that is enough.

If you don't feel that there is any one person that can be a solid support for you, especially in the first four to six months of embarking on your new path, it can be a great idea to seek other individuals or groups with similar goals, or even to hire a personal coach.

The good news is that support is not strictly limited to people, as I mentioned above. A healthy combination of a few good supportive people and your own personal support systems should help to keep you moving in a forward direction, no matter what challenges cross your path.

Places

· · · · · ·

Where do you feel at your best? Identify these places, and then make a point to spend more time there! Your physical environment can also have a huge influence on your mood and motivation. To support your commitments to yourself, plan to spend more time in the places that enforce your strengths and help you to deepen your connection to yourself and your true desires. This may be out in nature, or in a dedicated space in your home.

Wherever these places are for you, plan to spend time in at least one of them for at least half an hour each day—and commit to this time in your agenda book.

It's equally important to identity the places where you *don't* feel uplifted, inspired, and strong, and to make a point to avoid these. This applies to all areas of your life—where you live, work, work out, and spend leisure time.

For example, if you feel uncomfortable and self-conscious at your gym, it may be time to find another fitness facility or another form of activity altogether. There are so many ways to stay fit besides going to the gym. Or if your lunchroom at work always has doughnuts or other tempting, unsupportive foods that may thwart your efforts (especially in the beginning of your journey), you may need to choose another location to enjoy your lunch hour.

Until your new supportive habits have become deeply engrained, it's possible that the wrong environments will bring you down, throw you off track, or, even worse, trigger a reversion to old unsupportive beliefs and habits. Devote some time to making "places I love" and "places I avoid" lists—and honor these as boundaries, for the sake of your self-care and self-worth.

Passions

. . . .

What gives you joy, pleasure, excitement, or a sense of purpose?

The problem for many people when they take on new lifestyle changes is they forget that the process is also meant to be enjoyable! They look at it only as a short-term "fix"—especially with food and fitness—after which they can get back to life as usual and have fun again (this is the diet cycle).

But if the process of getting there isn't fun (whatever "fun" means to *you*), what are the chances that you'll be able to maintain your momentum over the long term? Probably very small.

So whatever it is that you've set out to do, make it fun, dammit!

In other words, don't get a gym membership if you don't like the gym. (I'm speaking from experience here—I've donated to many a gym establishment in the past.) But if you love to dance, run, swim, bend and twist, punch and kick, paddle, skate, bike, jump, ski, climb, or even walk… there's *probably* something else out there for you.

Don't commit to eating kale every day if you can't stand the taste of it (although I do recommend giving it a chance). Last time I checked, there were plenty of other vegetables to choose from in the produce section.

Here's another biggie: don't commit to creating elaborate healthy meals every day if you hate spending time in the kitchen (or if you don't have time, and it would only end up frustrating you). There are many ways to eat healthy without having to devote half your life to cooking. (I even have a special tip to help with this in Step Eight.) But if you're passionate about cooking, of course, by all means, go for it!

This, I believe, is a huge missing link for so many people. They hear that they "should" do something for their health or weight loss, and then they get down on themselves when they don't have the "discipline" to just do it. I know I've mentioned this a few times already, but just in case you missed it—*there's more to maintaining a healthy lifestyle than just discipline.* So much more. I learned this myself after many, many years of starting and unsuccessfully following through on many, many things that I "should" have done. I'd be willing to bet that if what you are doing doesn't match *your passions*, it's not going to stick or make you happy— even if it gives you short-term results.

When you begin to get clear on what you really love to do, your new supportive behaviors will be in alignment with *you*, which is a much more sustainable and enjoyable approach for the long term.

If you still need a little more convincing, remember the Law of Attraction? Well, if you shiver at the thought of dragging your butt to the gym, then working out will become something negative that you always dread doing. But if it makes you smile because you love the feeling of getting a good sweat on and socializing at the same time, then it will be something you are much more likely to do. Choosing only activities that you love will help you to think about working out in a much more positive light and to attract more opportunities to do them.

Here are a few examples from my own journey:

For starters, I've learned that I'm an introvert at heart, and the last thing I want to do is make small talk with someone while waiting for a weight machine. So, over the years, I've discovered that the activities that work best for me involve flying solo or at least being in enforced silence. Activities like yoga, running, swimming, and intense-interval workout DVDs in my living room suit me very well.

I know I can push myself hard on my own, focus on my breath, and not have to worry about using precious energy on socializing. I also find these activities meditative (with the exception of my workout DVDs), so they provide me with more than a physical benefit, too. *All* of the activities that I've chosen to incorporate into my life bring me joy. I love them and it's easy both to schedule them into my planner and to actually do them. But if I'd scheduled "go to the gym," I swear I'd be making every excuse in the book to delay or avoid it.

I'm also a nutritionist who seriously dislikes spending more than half an hour in the kitchen preparing a meal—unless it's for a special occasion. I like simplicity. I like healthy, delicious, and no-fuss meals—a combination that's entirely possible, I realize now.

> Consult your internal "joy guides" first, before you go looking for external guidance.

But my experience every time I tried to start a new diet plan was one of pure frustration because I would be spending many more hours than I ever wanted to in the kitchen. I preferred to be doing other things, but since I really wanted to follow the diet plans accurately, I would make this sacrifice. Then I would resent it; even if the food tasted good, I would rarely enjoy it because of all the time it took to prepare. And of course, I never lasted for more than a week on any diet, as typical menu plans offer plenty of lovely new recipes to try *every day of the week*. A sure failure waiting to happen for yours truly.

So, I encourage you, before you go looking for external guidance (which is still very helpful and important), to consult your internal "joy guides" first. Your Forever Body depends on it.

Step Five Actions Checklist

☐ *Preparation:* Start a vision or dream board (maybe even host a vision-board party!).

☐ Get yourself an agenda book or planner *that you love* and fill in activities for this month.

☐ Identify your support tools: equipment, clothing, food/ ingredients, etc. Start collecting the necessities.

☐ Identify your personal support systems to keep you on track—and set them up!

☐ *People:* Identify and enlist your support team.

☐ *Places:* Identify your supportive places and schedule time there (in your planner) each day.

☐ Identify the people and places you also want to avoid.

☐ *Passions:* Identify what's fun for you, what you love that will drive positive behaviors and habits. Make a list of possible activities that can fulfill this drive and support you in your goals.

"In the process of letting go, you will lose many things from the past, but you will find yourself."

DEEPAK CHOPRA

Step Six:
Let Go

. . . . .

AT THIS POINT in the process, it's important to pause and take a close look at some limitations that you could be unknowingly hanging onto that can definitely slow or even halt your progress.

There are five key things I believe everyone needs to let go of in order to achieve a Forever Body for good. Here they are, in no particular order:

Old Beliefs and Old Ways of Doing Things

During your journey, you may find how you used to do things may have held you back. Let go of rigidity and be open to new ways of thinking and acting. You may be surprised by a solution that you never thought might be feasible for you.

In my case, I had to give up my belief that I wasn't an "athlete" because I wasn't naturally good at sports. I always thought that the best way for me to manage my weight and physique was to monitor my food intake carefully and to do things like yoga and walking—activities that were noncompetitive and didn't require much athletic ability.

Even though I *loved* those activities and still do, I've realized over time that I actually do have some athletic genes in my body (and I believe that everyone does—you just have to find the right "sport" for you). Since then, I've been able to ramp up my fitness to peak levels and develop muscles that I never thought I was genetically designed to have because I let go of my old limiting belief.

> Let go of rigidity and be open to new ways of thinking and acting. You may be surprised by a solution that you never thought might be feasible for you.

I found that I love cardiovascular activities like swimming and running. These sports fuel my energy and spirit, and with practice (surprise, surprise), I could do them quite well. Although weight training never really stuck with me, despite many attempts to start programs over the years, I discovered there were other ways to build up strength, including short and effective HIIT workouts and Ashtanga yoga (an intense form of yoga that combines my love of movement, mindfulness, and balance, with challenging my muscles in new ways every time I hit the mat).

I also changed my belief that I could get everything I needed nutritionally from my diet alone, without taking supplements. I became open to shifting this belief as I learned, through my education, that it's just not possible for most of us to get everything we need nutritionally from our food (especially if we don't grow all our own food and have a good understanding of the quality of the soil we grow it in). Supplementation is not only recommended; it's essential. When I added supplements to my diet and started getting more of what my body was missing, I experienced incredible changes in my energy, mood, and immune system (and even my skin, hair, and nails). I've been able to tap into my body's natural energy sources (and "happy" hormones), so I can function without caffeinating myself, which before I never thought was possible. (I used to believe that coffee was essential to life itself—now I drink it because I love the taste, not because I need it.)

Are you holding on to some outdated beliefs that could be limiting your options—and hence your progress? There are way too many examples of unsupportive beliefs I could mention here, but here's a classic example:

"Self-care is selfish." Maybe you haven't said it out loud, but if you put others' needs before your own, this is most likely a limiting underlying belief. Could you be open to a new, empowering belief? How about "putting my self-care first allows me to give my best to others"?

Another great example of a limiting belief, particularly for those who love an active social life, is "I can't stick to my diet in social settings." Do you see how this might be totally out of alignment with your values? Would you be open to letting that go and replacing it with something more supportive to a sustained healthy lifestyle? How about "I surround myself with positive people who support me in living a life of joy and vibrant health."?

Shifting your beliefs—letting go of old, limiting ones and being open to new, supportive ones—can open up a whole new world of possibilities for you, your body, and your life.

Fear

· · · · ·

What is there to be afraid of when we're trying to lose weight or get fit? I believe that *fear of success* is a very real thing, for women especially and particularly when it comes to releasing extra weight.

Fear is our mind's way of protecting us from harm and keeping us safe. It can be a good thing sometimes—activating our "fight or flight" response so we stay alive—but, most often, the things we're afraid of are imagined outcomes. And we can be unaware of them, unless we take a closer look...

What will happen when you release the extra weight for good? We've already looked at the positive side (solidifying your commitment in Step Three); here we examine what's (falsely) portrayed as the negative side. There are so many possible answers to this question that it's difficult for me to highlight every one, but here are some examples of possible fears to explore:

- Is this extra weight something that you've been holding on to for so long that it's become part of your identity? (That is, are you afraid of losing your identity?)

- Is it your excuse for not taking on bigger projects or feeling deserving of love? (That is, are you afraid of "putting yourself out there" in personal and professional endeavors or relationships?)

- Is it your shield, your protection? (That is, are you afraid of being "exposed," being vulnerable, or being noticed?)

- Is it familiar and comfortable? (That is, are you afraid of change?)

When I reflect on my own journey—as I continued to gain weight when I was trying to lose it and get fit—I now see that my resistance to (that is, my underlying fear of) achieving my goals was a fear of being judged for how my body looked. I attribute this to my modeling experience, where I was completely reliant on my looks for acceptance. So, although I *thought I wanted* to lose the weight to feel beautiful and successful, there was a conflicting fear-based resistance coming from wanting to be successful and loved even if I didn't achieve my "ideal" weight. This internal conflict was reflected in my actions.

Although I'm a *huge* proponent of feeling worthy of love and acceptance no matter our shape or size, I also realize that holding onto my old *fear* of being judged by my body (good or bad) contributed to a heck of a lot of self-sabotage—even in my simplest efforts to lead a healthier lifestyle.

Is any of this ringing true for you, as well? I bet if you did some soul-searching and identified what your current body size, shape, and/or composition means to you, you might discover some subconscious reservations about changing it for good, which could be causing you to self-sabotage, too.

The first step in letting go of fear is to name it: When you think about succeeding at this goal, what fears come up for you? Be as specific as you can—going deeper into each one until you get to its root.

The next step, based on my own experience, is to learn to laugh at it! When we lay it all out for ourselves and get crystal clear on exactly what fears have been holding us back, we can often see the ridiculousness in them. They're usually not life-threatening, and sometimes they're so simple and subtle that we can't imagine we've allowed them to hold us back for so long.

You may even want to have a little cry over that first . . . but then, if you can allow laughter to take over, this can be very empowering. Especially if shared with a close friend or partner, laughter about unnecessary fears can help you take back control, rendering them powerless for good.

The Idea That You Have "Failed" Before

Even if, in the past, you have "quit" one or many diet or fitness programs, know that you have not failed. If you are reading this book, and you have come this far in the process, you are still committed to yourself and your health. That means you haven't quit, and you definitely haven't failed. You just haven't found the right solution for you yet. That's all. The only way to truly fail at improving your health and your life is to give up trying, to give up the search—and I don't believe that most humans are designed to do this. We're solution seekers; we're problem solvers. That's why the weight-loss industry is the giant that it is: we're always searching!

Remember, also, that with each and every avenue we explore, there are lessons to be learned. You've probably learned more about your likes and dislikes, what works for you and what doesn't, how you most like to be supported, what skills you develop easily and what's more challenging for you. I certainly did. And as long as you're learning, you're not failing. You're simply on your own journey and the more you can apply the lessons you've learned, letting go of the idea that you've "failed," the more you'll be able to accelerate your results.

> As long as you're learning, you're not failing.

Comparisons

. . . .

Remember that there is absolutely no one—I repeat, no one—on this planet who is going through, and who has been through, the exact same situation as you and who has the exact same set of skills, limitations, and genetics as you do. Your situation—which includes your body (shape, biochemistry, and physiology), your life circumstances, your gifts and your strengths—is entirely unique to you. Your successes and setbacks cannot be fairly compared to anyone else's, in a good or bad way. Even comparing yourself to your old self is not encouraged, because you are a different person today than you were then.

This one has been a particularly "sticky" thing for me to let go of—as it started for me so early in life. When I look back now to my "fat thighs" insecurities at three years old, I can safely identify it as a case of early-onset *comparison syndrome*.

I was a healthy, active kid (who also happened to love mac and cheese, and white bread and processed-cheese sandwiches), and I was in no way fat, but in comparison to my older, tinier stepsister, I believed that I was.

I was also very shy and insecure as a child, and since my stepsister was more confident and outspoken than I was, I naturally believed that being more like her was my path to approval and acceptance. I've spent my entire adult life learning to tame this comparison syndrome, which is often accompanied by perfectionism and being extremely hard on myself. I still work to manage it every day.

In fact, I don't think it will ever be totally handled (since it applies to many other areas of life, not just my image). But

I constantly keep myself in check to ensure that I'm letting this go as quickly as it creeps in. I remind myself daily to look to others for inspiration, not comparisons, and to focus on my own strengths and journey.

To go back to my marathon analogy (from Step Four), when we're going for our personal best, and running our own race, the worst thing we can do is look sideways for comparison's sake. There may be others on the same road, but they're *not* running the same race as you. They're running their own.

As I ran my marathon last year, I couldn't help but notice all the different bodies, shapes, fitness levels, and ages of the participants. By the time I'd reached the start line, and knew what it had taken (in training and commitment) for each one of those runners to even get there, every single one of them was a hero to me. The pros, the first-timers (like me), the old-timers, and the take-their-timers—*all* of them were there to run their own race to the finish line and do the very best they could, given where they were physically, emotionally, and mentally on that particular day. (I happened to be struggling with knee pain for over half the marathon—which had never occurred in my training. So I found myself having to adjust my running, and my expectations, accordingly.)

Because of the immense physical strain this kind of race has on the body, we need to consistently tune in to our body's cues and needs, and adjust as we go. Everyone who reaches the start line in a marathon—whether they cross the finish line this time or next time or never—is amazing. It's entirely an individual race, and an individual experience.

As is finding your Forever Body.

Judgment

· · · · · · · · · · ·

It's human nature to want to judge, to form a personal opin-ion (whether expressed or not) about how things or people "should" be, look, or act. But when we get into the habit of judging others, it also becomes easy to judge ourselves (probably harshest of all) for not doing, eating, or spending our time or money on what we "should."

What happens when we don't do what we think we "should" be doing? We feel guilty. And when it comes to achieving what we want, guilt can be a highly disruptive emotion.[32]

For your most productive and enjoyable journey, let go of the word "should"—when referring to others, but espe-cially when referring to yourself. If you've done the work in the first five steps, this will be much easier to do. And when you've solidified your commitment, "I should" will most likely be replaced by "I will" anyway.

Replace judgment with compassion and kindness, and simply honor the journey that you, and others, are on. We're all here to learn our own lessons and fulfill our own dreams—and not everyone will share the same opinions about what these are!

I personally believe that for us to start seeing real change in industry standards regarding beauty, women especially need to start supporting instead of judging each other. What are our judgments and opinions usually based on, anyway? Norms? Standards? Aren't these the "rules" that we'd like changed?

The less we judge, the more we can start to celebrate each other for our differences and unique gifts and strengths. We can honor and accept ourselves and others for exactly where we are in our own journeys, right now.

Step Six Actions Checklist

. . . .

- ☐ Identify any unsupportive beliefs that may be limiting your progress and develop new, supportive beliefs to replace them.

- ☐ Identify any fears that may be sabotaging your efforts, and have a good laugh at them (and possibly a good cry).

- ☐ Think of a time when you thought you "failed" before, and make note of at least five lessons you learned from that experience. (You can probably find even more.) How can you apply those lessons to this process now?

- ☐ When you find yourself in comparison mode, go back to the work you did in Step Two (Love What You've Got) to remind yourself of your gifts and strengths, and find inspiration in others without comparing yourself to them.

- ☐ Stop your judgments (of yourself and others) in their tracks, and consciously replace them with compassion and kindness. Offer someone a genuine compliment, and notice the difference it can make. Do this for yourself, too.

- ☐ Let all that shit go, and keep letting it go—this is a daily work in progress!

> *"The mind's first step to*
> *self-awareness must be through the body."*
> GEORGE A. SHEEHAN

Step Seven:
Do Your Hunger Homework

· · · · ·

HERE'S WHAT MOST people do when they diet: they count things and measure out portions. And guess what? That may work for a short period of time, but for most people this is tedious and annoying, and it's a lot of work that seemingly has no end. (Do you seriously want to be "counting" forever??) Inevitably, this leads them to quit.

Statistically, 95 percent of dieters quit doing what may work for them over a short time and go back to old habits, especially after achieving their goal. I believe that one of the most detrimental aspects of diets is that they encourage us to rely completely on external sources to tell us what, when, and how much to eat. This leads people to tune out their bodies' own hunger and satiety cues, to the point where they can no longer function on their own without a diet. That was certainly my experience.

The best menu plan in the world won't work for even the most disciplined people over the long term! Following strict plans is boring, unsustainable, and not the way any-one really wants to *live*. Let's face it, dieting is not living. It's painful. And until we learn to be completely independent eaters—by tuning into our body's own needs—we will always be looking to diets to help us and we will be stuck in the painful cycle.

The most critical thing to learn about food and your body cannot be found in a menu plan.

Knowing when you are hungry enough to eat (but not too hungry) and full enough to stop eating (but not too full) is one of the most important things to learn, or rather relearn, if you want sustainable results. Menu plans don't tell you how to do this.

We are *all* born with the innate ability to know when and how much to eat—we actually have specific hormones whose sole functions are to give us these cues. (Babies pick up these cues effortlessly: crying when they're hungry and pushing away the boob when they're full.) But somehow, through our lives, we begin to "unlearn" how to listen to them—usually beginning with dieting. Luckily, there's an easy method for becoming reacquainted with our body's cues.

This is what I call your "Hunger Homework": learning how to recognize when you're hungry and when you're full—and how to listen to and act on the cues!

First, you need to become familiar with the hunger scale,[33] a scale of 1 to 10, which you use to rate your hunger or fullness:

1. **Starving**—you feel weak and grumpy (aka "hangry")
2. **Uncomfortably hungry**—you could eat everything in sight
3. **Very hungry**—your mind is preoccupied with food

4. **Hungry**—you feel the urge to eat
5. **Not hungry, not full**—you are thinking about things other than food
6. **Satisfied**—you could eat more, but you're no longer hungry
7. **Full but comfortable**—you could be sustained for three to four hours
8. **Too full**—you feel like you ate more than you needed
9. **Uncomfortably full**—you are starting to experience indigestion (and possibly serious gas...)
10. **"Thanksgiving" full**—you are unbuttoning your pants and getting ready for a nap

The next thing to do is to start journaling or tracking your levels of hunger (before eating) and fullness (after eating). If you're already using the *Food, Fitness, and Sleep Tracker* (www.FindingYourForeverBody.com/Resources), this can be an easy add-on to tracking your meals. Do this for at least a week, every time you eat, and you'll start to notice patterns.

For example, if you're waiting until you're at a 1 or 2 before you eat, most likely that's when you'll stop at a 9 or 10 (counterproductive to the goal, obviously). A good target to aim for is to consistently eat when you reach a hunger level of 3 or 4, and to stop eating when you'd rate yourself between 6 and 7 (or 8 if it's delicious and totally worth it!). This is how you will naturally start to build confidence and trust in yourself as an expert of *you*.

Eventually, you won't need to write anything down. As you learn to truly listen to and trust your body on a regular basis, it will become something you do automatically (again) and you won't need to even think about it anymore.

But What about Trusting Your Body with *What* to Eat?

That's another skill that will come with time, and with your commitment to eating more whole, natural (unprocessed, unrefined) foods, which will naturally reduce false cravings for things your body doesn't really need, like refined sugars and excess sodium. You'll discover through your exploration and tracking process that the best food choices for *you* are the ones that make you feel the best during and after eating and that give you the most energy.

The Role of Sleep

Sleep has a critical role in the successful application of your Hunger Homework. Have you ever noticed that after a good night's sleep, it's much easier to tune into your body and make more supportive choices—of food and other things—throughout the day?

There's actually a scientific reason for this: the hormones that control your hunger (ghrelin) and fullness (leptin) go completely out of whack when you aren't getting sufficient quality sleep. Ghrelin increases and leptin decreases—not exactly a great combination when trying to make more supportive choices.

When these hormones are out of balance, we tend to eat a whole lot more than our bodies actually need, and more often. We also tend to have more, and give in more easily to, cravings for energy-dense, high-sugar, and highly caffeinated foods and drinks.

In other words, when we're sleep-deprived, we can't tune into our natural signals, no matter how skilled we've become at understanding them. And millions of North Americans are walking around sleep-deprived every day.[34]

How can you start to prioritize sleep so that you can do your Hunger Homework successfully? Well, again this requires getting to know *your* body and its needs, but here are seven helpful guidelines that you can start with:

1. Get to know your body's best sleep times.

There is no single perfect sleep schedule for everyone. Maybe you're a night owl or a morning person. Most people know their best, most productive hours of the day—so it's up to you to determine the sleep schedule that best supports it. If you're reaching for caffeine and sugar all day for energy, and overeating in general, this is a good indication that the schedule you're currently maintaining may not be working for you. To figure out what *your* best hours of sleep are, it may help to keep a written log of your sleep times for a while (in your *Food, Fitness, and Sleep Tracker*). Experiment with different sleep and rise times, until you find a schedule that consistently makes you feel well rested.

Find your own rhythm and go with it—other people's opinions don't matter. (That is, if you're a night owl, don't let the opinions of those cheerful morning people get to you!) The only thing that matters is that you feel refreshed, rested, and restored when you wake up from your slumber.

2. Practice good sleep hygiene.

What's sleep hygiene? It's basically the collection of habits that you practice in the evenings to accommodate a good night's sleep. Here are some that work for most people:

- Turn off electronics and avoid screen time one hour before you go to sleep; this includes TV, computers, phones, and tablets. They're too stimulating and can keep you awake when you try to fall asleep (reducing your total sleep time), no matter how tired you are.

- Keep electronics out of the bedroom. Anything that can emit light or cellular/Wi-Fi signals may interfere with sleep quality.

- Have a bedtime routine: wash face, brush teeth, shower/bathe, read, meditate, journal, bedtime snack, etc. We know that kids thrive on this, as it mentally prepares them for bed, but so do adults.

- Supplement with natural (nondependent) sleep remedies, if needed.

3. Don't exercise close to bedtime.

I've found that finishing exercise at least three hours before scheduled sleep time is a good rule of thumb. If you have to choose between exercise and sleep (because you can't exercise earlier), choose sleep. It's *that* important. However, exercising at the right time for you, earlier in the day, *can* help to promote a better night's sleep (it enhances our "deep sleep" phase), so do what you can to get in at least a short workout earlier. Bottom line: exercise is recommended for good sleep, but it's best if done earlier in the day so you're not overly stimulated too close to your ideal sleep time.

4. Make the room as dark as possible during sleep hours.

Light can affect your body's natural rhythms—even if detected through your eyelids. So, if there's artificial light in your bedroom (either from an alarm clock, night-light, or street lamp), it may help your quality of sleep significantly to get rid of it and blacken your room completely. Cover the alarm clock, unplug the night-lights, close the door(s), and get some blackout blinds. You'll be amazed at how much of a difference this can make.

5. Invest in a good-quality pillow.

Your pillow should be well suited for your head and preferred sleep position, and it should support your neck properly. Discomfort from having the wrong pillow can be one of the biggest inducers of night wakings.

6. If you wake up in the night, don't panic.

The more you focus on how little time is left before the morning, the less likely you'll be able to fall back asleep. Instead, if you find yourself wide awake in the night, and

• •

You can also look at this as a wonderful opportunity to write down the dreams you were having before you woke up. Often, our subconscious minds communicate thoughts, ideas, and feelings to us through our dreams, so if you can capture them as you remember them, you can examine the meaning further—either right away, or the next day when you're more mentally alert. It's not very often that we get the opportunity to remember and analyze our dreams, so if you can reframe your mid-night wakings into opportunities to receive guidance from your dream interpretations, then you'll be much more relaxed about the lost sleep and you'll be able to fall back into your dreams much faster.

your mind starts working, get out of bed and write down the things that you're thinking about.

7. Write before bed.

If your mind is preoccupied or stressed about something, spend a few minutes before bed writing out your thoughts. Keeping a journal and getting your thoughts, ideas, or fears out on paper will help to reduce the chances of you waking up in the night thinking about these same thoughts, ideas, and fears. In fact, writing out problems has been known to help trigger your subconscious mind to start seeking solutions—even if you can't consciously think of them right away. (So don't be surprised if, after doing this a few times, you actually wake up the next morning with some clarity about your solutions and next steps!) This activity can promote reduced stress over the long term, and as a result, better, more consistent sleep.

Step Seven Actions Checklist

- ☐ Do your Hunger Homework for at least one week—until you can start to recognize and tune into your body's natural cues for when you're hungry enough to eat (3 to 4) and full enough to stop (6 to 7).

- ☐ Prioritize sleep—apply the seven tips for a good night's rest.

- ☐ Use your *Food, Fitness, and Sleep Tracker* for easy tracking of Hunger Homework and sleep.

*"The most important thing is to enjoy your life—
to be happy—it's all that matters."*

AUDREY HEPBURN

Step Eight:
Treat Yourself—
and Cheat—Daily

· · · · ·

TREATING (OR REWARDING) yourself and "cheating on your diet" are two concepts that I feel have been sabotaging the efforts of dieters for decades. And it's time to reframe them, once and for all, so that they can instead become empowering tools that actually benefit you along your journey.

Here's what's wrong with the way these terms are currently used, when it comes to dieting, weight-loss, or healthy lifestyle efforts: they encourage a deprivation mindset.

For example, treating or "rewarding" yourself with a piece of cake for going to the gym keeps you in the mindset that food can only be pleasurable when it's been "earned." "Cheating" is used to describe what happens when you eat that piece of cake and you haven't "earned" it. Both can cause people to quit their diet or health program altogether.

I want to help you reframe these terms so that they are no longer associated with deprivation, and they can instead bring more fun and pleasure to your Forever Body journey. The more you use them, the better your results will be! How's *that* for a mindset shift? Let's dive into both of these deeper now.

Treating Yourself

Half the fun of having a goal is treating or rewarding yourself when you achieve it, or take action toward it, right? Well, I personally don't think so. Not anymore.

In fact, I don't even like to use the word "reward" at all when it comes to achieving physical goals—because it implies that the thing you're doing (achieving a health goal) isn't rewarding enough itself.[35] And as we covered in Step Three, a Forever Body SMART goal should be Rewarding, even without the promise of an additional payoff.

If you are indeed going after a SMART goal and taking baby steps toward it every day, the *true reward* is the sense of accomplishment you get from bringing yourself closer to, and eventually achieving, your desired outcome. If the thought of achieving your goal doesn't feel rewarding enough for you, then it may be time to go back to Step Three and reestablish a goal that *is* rewarding for you.

I do, however, believe that it's extremely important to treat ourselves along the way. In fact, I'm a huge fan of treats—on a daily basis! I believe that giving yourself a steady stream of fun, pleasurable experiences to balance out the discipline and consistent effort that you're investing into your progress is an incredibly important part of sustaining your efforts and maintaining your results over the long term. In my experience, regular treats can indeed help keep your energy, spirits, and motivation high—because they keep your well filled.

But *only* if you treat yourself without guilt. This is where we need to distinguish what a *real treat* is for *you*. Too often, the word "treat" gets associated with food. But for a Forever Body lifestyle, it's best if you can separate your food choices from your treats.

> Give yourself a steady stream of fun, pleasurable experiences to balance out the discipline and consistent effort, and you'll sustain your efforts and maintain your results over the long term.

Food is a necessity of life, not a treat. It's important that we balance out our food choices to include those that are nourishing for both body and soul. When we do this—when we really consider the food that we're about to eat and consciously choose to eat it—then we can avoid feelings of guilt around food.

If you follow the 80/20 rule most days, you won't ever need to consider food as a "treat." All foods will simply become part of your balanced lifestyle: 80 percent of the time, choose high-quality, high-nutrient foods and, during the other 20 percent, choose foods that you might have otherwise considered "treats"—and choose them wisely.

I personally like to evaluate these foods for their "worth-it-ness": that is, if the pleasure (taste, comfort, etc.) of eating them is, without question, worth claiming a portion of my precious 20 percent, then I eat it. If it only scores a "meh," then I don't. It's that simple. When you're never depriving yourself, and when you're consuming only moderate portions of the less-nutritious options only 20 percent of the time, you'll maintain your efforts so much more easily. And when 80 percent of your food intake is nutrient-dense, your body will be well equipped to avoid cravings and the other potentially negative effects of the other 20 percent.

Guilt is a very low-vibration (negative-energy) emotion,[36] and I personally believe that if we project that negativity onto our food as we're eating it, we're in fact consuming, digesting, and absorbing the negative energy along with it. This could be a huge source of indigestion, stress, and inflammation.

But when we consciously choose our food, eat it mindfully, appreciate every morsel, and allow our taste buds to relish the flavors, we will digest that food with ease. That's been my experience, and I stand strongly behind the belief that guilt is the greatest barrier to having a healthy relationship with food and our bodies. So, the more we can do to eliminate it, the easier it is to embrace and maintain our Forever Bodies.

So, if food isn't considered a treat, what is?

Again, this is individual, and it involves identifying the "treats" that fuel you, energize you, lift your spirits, give you pleasure, and motivate you to keep going with your chosen actions each day. These could be scheduled activities, deliberate gifts for yourself, or simply a time slot each day for doing whatever the heck you want to do.

Perhaps it's going to a movie, buying yourself flowers or an uplifting essential oil, having a date with your significant other or coffee with a friend, taking a relaxing bath, getting a pedicure, or signing up for that dance class you've been dying to join forever. It can be anything that speaks to *you* and *your* personal energy needs. It could even be as simple as getting your partner to take the kids out for an afternoon so you can enjoy some quality alone time.

I love my alone time—particularly if I can spend it outdoors near the ocean. I used to think of taking a beach walk as a reward for getting things done, but now I consider it a daily treat, no matter how much I've accomplished, to reenergize and reconnect with myself. It fills me up, so why should I wait until I've "earned" it to allow myself that pleasure? When I do take the time to enjoy it, it gives me more fuel to get even more accomplished.

Make a list of as many feel-good (non-food) treats as you can think of. Be sure to include both large and very small ones—you'll want to enjoy both, though you may not have time for the larger ones every day. Then, determine how you will fit these into your day. Some of them may require planning (in your agenda book) and asking for support.

Do not delay your treats—if you go too many days without treating yourself to something fun and refueling, your well may run completely dry. That is precisely the time when most people reach for "comfort" foods or other comforting yet unsupportive behaviors (drinking, smoking, TV/social media binges...) to help them feel some short-term pleasure. But these behaviors always have negative repercussions—mostly on self-esteem and the belief that we can sustain our supportive efforts. I've found the best way to avoid getting into this state is to keep a constant drip flowing into your well—through daily, mandatory, guilt-free treats.

Note: I believe this is an absolute *must* for confidently maintaining your Forever Body. This is why a treat must never be associated with feelings of guilt. If you're feeling guilty about the time, money, or other resources required to treat yourself, then I urge you to examine why this is.

If you feel guilty about time—like there never seem to be enough hours in a day for regular responsibilities, let alone for taking your treats—then go back to the Planning section in Step Five and ensure that you're keeping a balanced schedule. Take a look at activities and commitments that you may be able to eliminate or decrease spending time on, in favor of your treat time. It's that important. This is an area of guilt that I'm personally *very* familiar with—I've always felt a sense of urgency around my other responsibilities, like household chores, mommy duties, and activities that keep my business rolling. But I've realized that if I don't make the time for myself, I'm much less effective and efficient at all of those things and I don't feel as good at the end of the day, even though I've accomplished tasks on my list. We *need* both: time for other priorities and time for self. And sometimes this means reprioritizing and eliminating less-important tasks for the sake of creating your most balanced and healthy lifestyle.

If you feel guilty about money—like you're going into debt by treating yourself—it may be the time to look at your budget and rework it so that you can actually allocate planned funds specifically for this purpose (10 percent of income[37] is a good amount to ensure that you never feel deprived, yet it won't break the bank). If the budget is still too tight, then choose treats that are effective yet inexpensive. It doesn't cost much to take a long bath or walk along the beach. It can also be fun to create your own home-spa experience with a few ingredients that go a long way—a foot bath, face mask, relaxing music, and essential oils can add up to a wonderful hour spent at home.

If you feel guilty about asking for help or support—like you don't want to burden others in order to treat yourself—then it may be time to take a close look at your "emotional bank accounts" with the people in your life. Are they depositing (giving) more than they're withdrawing (taking) from your account (relationship)? If so, how can you deposit more back into the relationship so that it becomes balanced?

> Balanced emotional accounts help to eliminate guilt.

Balanced emotional accounts help to eliminate guilt. You may also discover through this process that you've been depositing more than you've been withdrawing. In this case, it's fair to request withdrawals that will help to rebalance (and in most cases, help to heal) the relationships from which you're feeling the most guilt.

The bottom line is, if you don't make treating yourself a priority every day, no one else will. You deserve it, whether or not you feel you've "earned" it. Treats don't have to be earned; they are a basic human need that should not be ignored. They are indeed an integral part of your *joy*-filled, Forever Body journey.

Cheating

Why is it that so many people are afraid to "cheat" on their diets? I want to help you reframe cheating so that this worry becomes a thing of the past—and you can achieve success while "cheating on your diet," every single day.

First, let's look deeper into the real definition of cheating.

The *Oxford Dictionary* says to cheat is to "gain unfair advantage by deception or breaking rules."[38] Given this definition, how can eating unsupportive foods possibly be considered an advantage, fair or unfair, for achieving your health goals? To me, cheating is all about giving yourself an advantage—making your life, and your progress toward your goals, easier!

This concept of reframing cheating to use it to our advantage first came to me several months ago when a friend who knew I was working on this book asked me: "So, do you ever, like, cheat? You know... eat a hamburger, or ice cream, or something really, really bad?"

I thought about it for a moment and then answered: "Well, I do eat those things from time to time, but I never refer to it as cheating... anymore. I just call it 'keeping myself balanced.'"

Then, after another pause for thought, I continued. "I do 'cheat,' though. I find ways to eat super healthy without making complicated meals, growing my own food, or even spending that much time in the kitchen. For a nutritionist, I'm actually pretty lazy," I said, laughing. "I take a *lot* of shortcuts to stay incredibly healthy!"

What kind of shortcuts do I take to "cheat" my way to a healthy Forever Body? This is by no means a complete list of "cheats," but they're some of my favorites:

- I supplement daily (multivitamins, Essential Fatty Acids, probiotics, energizing/balancing herbs and greens, and some digestive enzymes, as needed).

- I buy my fresh greens pre-(triple)washed. If I buy a head of lettuce or bunch of greens and have to wash them myself, this significantly reduces my chances of consuming them.

- I even buy my fresh organic herbs in a tube! These are brilliant additions to the produce section.

- I make my best meals in a super-high-speed blender—smoothies, warm soups, and healthy desserts are my favorite go-to foods when I'm short on time, or when I'm feeling too lazy. No tedious chopping required!

- I buy organic, quality beans, soups, and sauces that are ready to open and heat in a pan in minutes. On the very odd occasion, I will actually spend hours in the kitchen preparing a meal from scratch on the stovetop—but this must be by choice, not necessity.

- I consume sprouted and fermented foods (great for gut health and digestion) all the time—and eat them with *everything*. Sauerkraut isn't just for sausages in my house!

- I spend a day or two every month doing a full-body herbal cleanse. I'm definitely not perfect, but I've learned the body is very forgiving when we give our hard-working organs and cells the rest and support they deserve.

That's how I cheat! I have a ton of other activities I like to spend my time doing, other than cooking in the kitchen. So whenever I can shorten my time spent in that room, I do.

This cheating philosophy can be applied to fitness, too! Twenty-to-thirty-minute high-intensity and effective workouts could help you cheat your way to a healthy, fit body, so you don't have to spend hours at the gym. Adding in some post-workout nutrition, like a *high-quality* sports nutrition shake, can also speed up the process. I'm "guilty" of both these fitness cheats.

In a perfect world, we'd all be growing our own veggies, milking our own cows, and raising our own hens right in our backyards, with the best organic feed and soil, in order to live the healthiest lives possible. But that's just not realistic for most of us. Most of us need to "cheat" our way to a healthy lifestyle. We need to find ways to make maintaining a healthy diet and lifestyle easy and sustainable. And that's what I encourage you to begin examining for yourself. (*Note*: I'm *not* encouraging or endorsing weight-loss or appetite-suppressing supplements—those are definitely not supportive of a Forever Body.)

In what areas of your lifestyle—food, fitness, or otherwise—do you feel you need to find support shortcuts? Maybe you'll get some ideas from my list, and even seek out your own. Be creative and find what works for you. Maybe there's even an app for that!

When it comes to achieving your Forever Body, there is never any shame or guilt involved with this reframed definition of cheating. It simply means that you're ensuring your long-term success with as much ease and grace as possible.

Step Eight Actions Checklist

- ☐ Make a list of daily (small and big) treats you can indulge in to keep your mood and motivation high.
- ☐ Schedule one today.
- ☐ Make a "cheat" sheet of different ways you can make your healthy lifestyle and nutrition easier for you (use my free online *Nutrition Resource*, if needed: www.FindingYour ForeverBody.com/Resources).

> *"To truly cherish the things that are important to you, you must first discard those that have outlived their purpose."*
>
> MARIE KONDO

Step Nine:
Create Space

· · · · ·

HERE'S A VERY important lesson I've learned along my journey: it's extremely difficult, if not impossible, to invite permanent change when we're holding on to the things, situations, and even people in our lives that are no longer serving us.

They have "outlived their purpose" because they don't "fit" or support our vision and desires, and the longer we hold onto them, the more they can hold us back from our *real* desired outcome—and cause a ton of self-sabotage on our health goals in the process.

They are essentially clutter, which can cause excess, unnecessary stress and even depression if held onto for too long. When I look back at my turning point for the better, I can clearly see that addressing, and eliminating, the clutter in my life was a crucial step in driving me forward in a way I'd never been able to do before. And I can guarantee that your success with your health goals will be short-lived if your life is cluttered in other areas.

To welcome in a new *permanent* state of health and well-being, we need to create space for it. We need to clear out the clutter—both physically and emotionally.

How can you identify clutter? Think of the things in your life right now that cause you stress, zap your energy, dampen your mood, or steal your joy on a regular basis—but that you tolerate anyway. You "step over it" instead of picking it up and discarding it.

The clutter in your life can generally be divided into two categories: *physical clutter* and *emotional clutter*. Though they can be categorized differently, they are very much linked, as the physical clutter in our environments can be a useful gauge for the emotional clutter we're carrying.

> Your success with your health goals will be short-lived if your life is cluttered in other areas.

In other words, when we're weighed down by emotional clutter, this can manifest around us as physical clutter.

Physical clutter is anything in your personal environment (home, work space, car, etc.) that drives you crazy but that you've just learned to overlook or bypass. You know you want to change it, but you haven't had the motivation, time, or energy to do anything about it.

Emotional clutter is anything that causes excess stress in your life that drains your energy—perhaps a toxic relationship or stressful situation that is bogging you down. A certain amount of stress in day-to-day life is normal and natural, but when it becomes debilitating, that's when stress becomes clutter.

Both can be detrimental to your health goals and to achieving your desired vision for your future.

As I shared with you earlier, I had a *lot* of emotional clutter going on in my life (before my personal turning point—for the better). And when I looked around my home, it was clear:

- I rarely cleaned anymore.

- You couldn't see our bathroom counter for all the beauty products that were strewn across it.

- There was evidence *everywhere* of at least three different side businesses I'd explored and started.

- Our bedroom had become a dumping site for anything that I didn't want to deal with right away—and the door remained permanently shut.

Interestingly, when I look back, the biggest site of physical clutter (bedroom) in my life was a clear indication of the biggest source of my emotional clutter (my struggling marriage). No amount of "healthy eating" could make up for the drain that this had on my energy.

My personal example may be more extreme than most. Clearing my clutter meant a lot of *big* changes—which I didn't tackle all at once, but they weren't too far apart (they occurred within a two-year time frame). For me to create space for what I really wanted in my life, I let go of my job, my marriage, and my entire home (even my province!), which is not what I'm suggesting you do here.

I'm not requesting that you completely resolve *all* the clutter in your life at once. It is, however, important to begin acknowledging all the sources of clutter—both physical and emotional—and to think how you can address, and eventually eliminate them, one by one, over time.

There may be things that you've been tolerating *most of your life*. Although you know they're weighing down your spirit, you may feel as though they're too overwhelming or even impossible to change at the moment. But taking a closer look at the areas of your life that may be causing you unnecessary stress is indeed a critical step for optimal health and for finding your Forever Body.

Before I started dealing with the clutter in my own life, I always had very limited success with my health and fitness efforts. I struggled with staying motivated, I felt overwhelmed by time commitments, and I was depleted of my energy from dealing with all the stress.

When I began to address and eliminate sources of clutter in my life, particularly the emotional clutter, it gave me such a surge of energy and motivation that it made keeping my commitments to myself and my health (that is, my self-care) so much easier.

If it's so bad for us, why do we tolerate it? Why do we hold onto clutter when it's no longer serving us? The truth is, it's not easy. It can be sad to let go of things, situations, and people that are familiar, and change can be very, very hard. But living with clutter can be even harder. And heavy—very, very heavy.

Yes, tackling your emotional clutter can be very difficult and requires a lot of your energy in the short term, but I can say with 100-percent confidence that the eventual payoff to your body, mind, and soul is truly worth it in the long run.

Tackling the Clutter

I've noticed over the years that when I'm experiencing significantly more stress, the "tolerations" in my environment increase significantly, too. My external environment (my home, workplace, and car) is a mirror of what's going on in my internal environment. And what I've found is that, because the two are so connected, I can start to deal with my emotional clutter by tackling my physical clutter.

In other words, if I'm dealing with a stressful situation, and I take some time to clear out some tolerations in my environment, this actually gives me more mental and emotional energy and clarity to deal with the emotional stuff.

So the good news is that, no matter which one you choose to tackle first, the other will inevitably benefit. And physical clutter is by far the easiest one to start with.

Physical Clutter

Some people may be dealing with the prospect of a lot more physical clutter than others. So, if the idea of tackling the clutter in your environment feels overwhelming, I encourage you to take the same baby-step approach that you've begun to do with your other Forever Body goals. The important thing here is to just start. And don't quit.

A great way to begin is by simply making a list of all the tolerations in your environment. List the bigger items (for example, a messy home office), and choose *one* that you want to start working on right away.

Then, break that *one* big source of clutter down into smaller, manageable tasks (open mail, file papers, pay bills, dust keyboard, etc.). Once you've broken down the tasks, go through them one by one and either:

- do it (or schedule to do it, in your agenda book),
- delegate it, or
- outsource it.

If you're going to be doing or scheduling the tasks yourself, I highly recommend following some decluttering principles taken from Feng Shui.[39] They can make these tasks much less daunting and even easy. Here are the basics:

1. Spend a *maximum of 30 minutes at a time, no more than three times a week,* decluttering. Use your agenda book and use a timer—it's very important that you do not exceed this time. When the timer goes off, you are done until the next scheduled time.

2. Establish a good sorting system, especially if you have a lot of items to sort through (such as in closets or other cluttered spaces). Prepare four separate boxes and label them
   - keep,
   - throw away,
   - donate, and
   - I don't know.

You should be able to assign items to a box within seconds—if you have to pause and think about it for too long, put it in the "I don't know" box. Once your "I don't know" box is full, put it away in the basement or garage for six months; then, if you haven't opened it within that time frame, leave it sealed and just donate it.

It's also important that you don't just "keep" everything. If you're holding onto physical clutter, this is a limiting resistance to change, and it typically transfers to all areas of your life. If you're ready for change, let it go and make room for the new. Establish some clear guidelines for yourself to determine what you will keep, such as the following:

- I currently use it.
- I will use it within the next six months.
- It has sentimental value.

By ridding your environment of any unnecessary physical clutter *one* source and *one* task at a time, you will feel much lighter and more energized, which will contribute significantly to your momentum as you continue along your Forever Body journey.

Emotional Clutter

These are typically much bigger items to deal with, and this may or may not be the right time to deal with them. As you begin to feel healthier, stronger, and more energized, solutions to your emotional clutter may become clearer. Now may be a good time to at least acknowledge them and envision the ideal outcome or solution that you would like to create (which you can add to your vision board).

For the larger areas of emotional stress, it may be appropriate to enlist the support of a qualified coach or counselor to help you declutter when you're ready to take on the process of overcoming these issues. But for the smaller areas of emotional stress, there are some ways to start decluttering on your own, and daily.

It's important to have an outlet to declutter the toxic stress that accumulates each day and to also have some conscious strategies to prevent toxic overload. These outlets and strategies can be different for everyone, but here are some great, proven techniques that may work for you (I personally benefit from most of these, regularly if not daily):

- Meditate—and if you find meditation difficult, try a guided meditation (like my *Self-Talk Detox*) or a mild activity that helps clear your mind, such as yoga or walking.

- Keep a written journal to give your thoughts a practical voice and to record ideas and solutions.

- Engage in at least 30 minutes of cardiovascular exercise to help raise serotonin (the "happy" hormone).

- Talk it out with a good friend, loved one, or coach/counselor who can help to lift your spirits and support you in finding solutions.

- Evaluate your priorities and commitments and say no more often to honor your time and energy.

- Limit time on social media to reduce your propensity for comparisons, "taking on" bad news, and feeling guilty over time wasted.

- Avoid gossip and negativity, which tend to zap energy, decrease motivation, and drop mood.

- Express gratitude for the positive things in your life to lift mood, energy, and motivation (and to attract more positive things and solutions!).

Step Nine Actions Checklist

· ·

☐ List the sources of physical clutter in your environment.

☐ Choose *one* and break it down into smaller tasks.

☐ Add time to your planner to tackle them (30 minutes, three times a week), until complete. Repeat for other items on your list.

☐ Acknowledge areas of emotional clutter; create a vision of your future desired outcome (bonus: add it to your vision board as a reminder).

☐ Choose *one* strategy for reducing stress, and apply it daily.

"If you can dream it, you can do it."
WALT DISNEY

Step Ten:
Expand

. . . . .

No, I'm not referring to your body or waistline. This step is about expanding your mind.

Have you ever had the experience of *not focusing on your body, food, or your weight at all*, and yet somehow you lost weight during that time?

I hear it often. It comes in a variety of expressions. Here are some examples:

"I was so busy (with that project, event, etc.) that I didn't have time to fuss over my diet, and yet I was surprised to see the weight fall off."

"As I was falling in love, I ate whatever I wanted and I still lost weight."

"I enjoyed every day on my vacation without even thinking about my diet and I didn't gain a pound—in fact, I even lost some weight!"

There's a very good reason for all of these scenarios. They all have something very important in common—with each other and with my Personal French Paradox that I experienced briefly during my painful dieting days.

The focus was redirected to something bigger and more important in life.

Joy. Passion. Purpose. When we're feeling these emotions, we're in flow with our lives. Energy moves easily through us, and our bodies become our physical expression of these emotions. Food becomes less of a burdensome evil, and more of a life-sustaining necessity that can also provide pleasure.

But when we keep our focus narrowed onto the small, unimportant details like calories or the number on the scale, this can suck the joy, passion, and energy right out of our souls. So it's time to start focusing on the bigger, more important things in your life.

Achieving a Forever Body doesn't come from just focusing on your body!

There is a reason you were put on this planet, and it wasn't just to look good! Your mission in this lifetime is to figure out what that reason is. (Hint: feeling joy when you're engaged in something is a good sign that you're getting closer.) The great news is that you don't have to have the perfect butt:waist:boob ratio to start moving forward on your bigger passions and purpose.

Expand your vision. Focus on the things that really matter. What do you want to create in this lifetime? How do you want to be remembered? What do you want your legacy to be? Chances are, it's not your weight or your size. Think bigger than your physical body: Why are *you* here?

When you begin to shift your focus, expand your vision beyond simply what and how much you're eating each day, and start taking action in the direction you want to go, positive results in your physical body become a natural side effect of living joyfully and passionately.

Your vibrant health (not your size) is a *fundamental piece of your foundation* that will determine what you'll be able to do and create in this lifetime, and the difference you'll be able to make. When we're passionate about life, this naturally makes us motivated to keep our energy high by eating well and staying active. Nutrition, fitness, and self-care become the *means* to achieve other more important things in life—they are not the end goals.

What parts of your life do you need to start nurturing to bring you closer to your joy, passion, and purpose?

What relationships—including your relationship with yourself—do you need to devote more energy to?

What activities do you need to make more time for?

What education or training do you need to invest in to move forward in the direction of your passions and purpose?

What people do you need to spend more time with for inspiration and heart-warming connection?

What do you need to ask for (from people, God, or the universe) to bring you closer to fulfilling your purpose? (When we ask for the signs and/or the answers, they are usually provided to us in creative ways.)

When you start to expand on and live your vision each day, just one baby step at a time, you can recreate that feeling of falling in love and being on the best vacation, every single day. You can achieve your Forever Body as though you weren't even looking.

Step Ten Actions Checklist

· ·

☐ Ask the self-reflection questions: What do I want to create in this lifetime? How do I want to be remembered? What do I want my legacy to be?

☐ Add your vision to your vision board.

☐ Expand on your vision by identifying what support, education, training, actions—and even miracles—you will need to make your vision a reality.

☐ Identify the parts of your life, including relationships, you will need to nurture in order to start living your vision soon, if not right away. Commit some baby steps to your agenda book to support this.

☐ Enjoy the ride! Manifesting your vision may take time, so it will require your patience, persistence, and faith. Use the collection of tools you've developed in previous steps to support you.

Final Words

· · · · ·

By THIS POINT, I hope that I've helped you to see that a true Forever Body has nothing to do with perfection or even your body size or appearance, for that matter. Perfect adherence to the "perfect" diet isn't what the majority of us are after, nor is it that perfect number—on the scale, the dress tag, or the tape measure. None of those "achievements" is the key to happiness.

A true Forever Body is about progression—inside and out. And that journey is not about "getting better," but more about learning and growing in a direction that feeds our mind, body, and soul in the best way possible.

In other words, having a Forever Body means that we are in a continuous, dynamic discovery process that brings us closer to the fullest expression of *who* we really are. There is never an "end result" or final destination, because *who* we are is constantly evolving, and so are our bodies. So, if you've already begun your journey toward better mental, emotional, and physical health, you have in fact already achieved your Forever Body.

Now it's simply time to honor it by applying the lessons you learn along the way, to help you nurture and nourish it with more ease, so that it continues to evolve and support you as your vehicle to experience all the joy and wonder that your life has to offer.

Personally, I feel as though I only started living ten years ago. For 30 years prior to that, most days felt like a struggle, and truly "happy" days seemed fleeting and sparse. With my food and body-image struggles now in the distant past, I'm able to finally fully enjoy my life and all the adventure it brings. Where once there was anxiety, there's now excitement for the future, as my Forever Body continues to be the magnificent vehicle that will allow me to create, learn, and experience anything that my mind and soul crave (writing more books, running more races, frolicking on more beaches around the world with my daughter, building beautiful friendships, creating new workshops and courses . . . to name but a few!).

Though I still face challenges and stress, and not every day is full of laughter and joy, the difference now is that I have an unwavering feeling of contentment and inner peace, no matter what's going on, because I've developed a deep sense of purpose and alignment with my authentic self. I've learned that happiness isn't necessarily a state of consistent outer joy but rather a sense of being consistently connected to *who* we are.

So, for your most successful and enjoyable Forever Body journey, I leave you with these final words:

1. Continue to do your best each day with the information you have available to you, and make a commitment to learning a little more every day.

2. Focus on developing more expertise in *you* every single day: what *your* mind, body, and soul need to *thrive*.

3. Pour your energy unapologetically into your self-care, self-acceptance, and self-empowerment, so you can *live fully as the most authentic version of you.* That's the real key to happiness.

And that's not something you'll find in any diet book, ever.

Acknowledgments

· · · · ·

FOR AS LONG as I can remember, I've wanted to become a writer and I'm so grateful to all the people in my life who have inspired, encouraged, supported, mentored, and coached me through the years to help me finally write and publish my first book.

To my mom, Judy Hitchcock; my BFF, Krista Hare; my Mark; and my shining light of a daughter, Eve, who have all given me a steady stream of unconditional love and support, from the moment we met: Thank You.

To my friends, new and old, and my family, near and far, who have been part of my journey and sent me good wishes and words of encouragement along the way (you know who you are): Thank You.

To my dear friends Erika Anderson, Melanie O'Leary, Krista Thrasher, and my writing buddy Robert Millington, as well as my "seester" Rose Record, who took the time to read and review my draft work and provide support and encouragement throughout my writing process: Thank You.

To Geoff Affleck and to Chris Kyle, who have each been phenomenal coaches and mentors through my self-discovery and development as a writer and teacher in my field of work: Thank You.

To Chris Attwood, Janet Attwood, Marci Shimoff, and Geoff Affleck, as well as the heart-centered Enlightened Bestseller Mastermind community, who have inspired me, and continue to inspire me, to live a passionate life: Thank You.

To Joel Roberts and Heidi Roberts who whole-heartedly believed in me and motivated me to build the confidence to share my message on a larger scale: Thank You.

To Susan Friesen, Daniel Simmons, and the team at eVision Media, who make my life so much easier by supporting me through—and providing me relief from—my "challenged" relationship with technology so that I can share my message globally: Thank You.

To the Rockstar team at Page Two Strategies, who helped me to transform my draft manuscript into a beautifully published book that I'm proud to put on my shelf and that I'm excited to share with others. Jesse Finkelstein, Gabrielle Narsted, Peter Cocking, Carra Simpson, Lucy Kenward, and my sent-from-Heaven editor, Erin Parker, who made the process of polishing and refining my manuscript as enjoyable and easy as possible, and made every stage of the process feel like a dance: Thank You.

And to the modeling agent who sent me away for my imperfections but unknowingly launched me on my path toward full self-love and acceptance so I could become a positive role model to my daughter: a massive, sincere Thank You.

Endnotes
and Resources

· · · · ·

1. "Eating Disorder Statistics," Statistic Brain, research conducted October 1, 2015, accessed December 15, 2016, http://www.statisticbrain.com/eating-disorder-statistics; Traci Mann, A. Janet Tomiyama et al., "Medicare's Search for Effective Obesity Treatments," *American Psychologist* 62, no. 3 (April 2007): 220-33, doi: 10.1037/0003-066X.62.3.220. See http://www.dishlab.org/pubs/MannTomiyamaAmPsy2007.pdf; D. Neumark-Sztainer, M. Wall et al., "Why Does Dieting Predict Weight Gain in Adolescents? Findings from Project EAT-II: A 5-Year Longitudinal Study," *Journal of the American Dietetic Association* 107, no. 3 (March 2007): 448-55, https://www.ncbi.nlm.nih.gov/pubmed/17324664.

2. "Body Image Statistics," Statistic Brain, research conducted January 26, 2016, accessed December 15, 2016, http://www.statisticbrain.com/body-image-statistics.

3. Jeanne B. Martin, "The Development of Ideal Body Image Perceptions in the United States," *Nutrition Today* 45, no. 3 (May/June 2010): 98–110, doi: 10.1097/NT.0b013e3181e37f75.

4. "Body Image Statistics," Statistic Brain.

5. "Overweight and Obesity Patterns (BMI ≥25) for Both Sexes Adults (20+)," Institute for Health Metrics and Evaluation, University of Washington, accessed December 15, 2016, http://vizhub.healthdata.org/obesity. From 2013 stats: 50.6% Canadian women, 63.1% US women.

6. "Marketing to Women Quick Facts," Sheconomy, accessed December 15, 2016, http://she-conomy.com/facts-on-women.

7. Marsha Hudnall and Karin Kratina, *Disordered Eating in Active and Sedentary Individuals* (Champaign, IL: Human Kinetics Publishers, Inc., 2005): Textbook to accompany course: see http://www.hkeducationcenter.com/courses/OEC_Previews/hf-sn314_preview/index.cfm.

8. Victor Chan, "Women Can Come to the Rescue of the World," The Dalai Lama Center for Peace + Education blog, January 25, 2010, http://dalailamacenter.org/blog-post/western-women-can-come-rescue-world.

9. "Alumni Profile: Kimberley Record," Canadian School of Natural Nutrition, http://csnn.ca/about/alumni-profiles/kimberley-record/.

10. Martin, "The Development of Ideal Body Image Perceptions," *Nutrition Today*.

11. "Body Image Statistics," Statistic Brain.

12. Sarah E. Jackson, Andrew Steptoe et al., "Psychological Changes following Weight Loss in Overweight and Obese Adults: A Prospective Cohort Study." PLOS ONE 9, no. 8 (August 6, 2014): e104552, doi: 10.1371/journal.pone.0104552. See also "Losing Weight Won't Make You Happy," UCL News, August 7, 2014, accessed December 15, 2016, https://www.ucl.ac.uk/news/news-articles/0814/070814-Losing-weight-will-not-make-you-happy.

13. Michael L. Dansinger, Joi Augustin Gleason et al., "Comparison of the Atkins, Ornish, Weight Watchers, and Zone Diets for Weight Loss and Heart Disease Risk Reduction: A Randomized Trial," Journal of the American Medical Association, 293, no. 1 (2005): 43–53, doi: 10.1001/jama.293.1.43, http://jamanetwork.com/journals/jama/fullarticle/200094.

14. "Number of American Dieters Soars to 108 Million," Marketdata on prweb, January 10, 2012, accessed December 15, 2016, http://www.prweb.com/releases/2012/1/prweb9084688.htm.

15. Charles Duhigg, *The Power of Habit: Why We Do What We Do in Life and Business* (Toronto: Anchor Canada, 2012), http://charlesduhigg.com/how-habits-work/.

16. James O. Prochaska, John C. Norcross, and Carlo C. DiClemente, Changing for Good: A Revolutionary Six-Stage Program for Overcoming Bad Habits and Moving Your Life Positively Forward (New York: HarperCollins, 1994): 133–36.

17. Paul S. MacLean, Audrey Bergouignan et al., "Biology's Response to Dieting: The Impetus for Weight Regain," *American Journal of Physiology—Regulatory, Integrative and Comparative Physiology* 301, no. 3 (September 1, 2011): R581–R600, doi: 10.1152/ajpregu.00755.2010, http://ajpregu.physiology.org/content/301/3/R581.

18. Craig Freudenrich, "How Fat Cells Work," HowStuffWorks.com, October 27, 2000, accessed December 15, 2016, http://science.howstuffworks.com/life/cellular-microscopic/fat-cell.htm.

19. Mayo Clinic Staff, "Liposuction," Mayo Clinic website, November 29, 2016, accessed December 15, 2016, http://www.mayoclinic.org/tests-procedures/liposuction/details/risks/cmc-20197277.

19. Virginia Lee Mermel cited in Marie Zahorick and Valeri Webber, "Postpartum Body Image and Weight Loss," La Leche League International website, accessed December 15, 2016, http://www.lalecheleague.org/nb/nbsepoct00p156.html.

21. Avinash De Sousa, "Towards an Integrative Theory of Consciousness: Part 1 (Neurobiological and Cognitive Models)," *Mens Sana Monographs* 11, no. 1 (January–December 2013): 100, doi: 10.4103/0973-1229.109335.

22. "What Is Law of Attraction?," Real Life Law of Attraction website, accessed December 15, 2016, http://www.real-life-law-of-attraction.com/what-is-law-of-attraction.html.

23. Carlos Augusto Monteiro, Renata Bertazzi Levy et al., "Increasing Consumption of Ultra-Processed Foods and Likely Impact on Human Health: Evidence from Brazil," *Public Health Nutrition* 14, no. 1 (October 25, 2010): 5–13, doi: doi: 10.1017/s1368980010003241, http://www.wphna.org/htdocs/downloadsdec2012/2011_PHN_Monteiro_et_al.pdf; Jean-Claude Moubarac, Ana Paula Bortoletto Martins et al., "Consumption of Ultra-Processed Foods and Likely Impact on Human Health. Evidence From Canada," *Public Health Nutrition* 16, no. 12 (November 2012): 1–9, doi: 10.1017/S1368980012005009, https://www.researchgate.net/publication/233745062_Consumption_of_ultra-processed_foods_and_likely_impact_on_human_health_Evidence_from_Canada; Dr. Joseph Mercola, "More than Half of the American Diet is Ultra-Processed Junk," Mercola website, March 23, 2016, accessed December 15, 2016, http://articles.mercola.com/sites/articles/archive/2016/03/23/ultra-processed-foods.aspx.

24. Mark Hyman, "How Malnutrition Causes Obesity," *The Huffington Post,* May 8, 2012, accessed December 15, 2016, http://www.huffingtonpost.com/dr-mark-hyman/malnutrition-obesity_b_1324760.html.

25. "Foods that Fight Inflammation," Harvard Health Publications, October 26, 2015, accessed December 15, 2016, http://www.health.harvard.edu/staying-healthy/foods-that-fight-inflammation.

26. Christian Nordqvist, "Food Intolerance: Causes, Symptoms, and Diagnosis," MNT, July 11, 2016, accessed December 15, 2016, http://www.medicalnewstoday.com/articles/263965.php.

27. Elson Haas and Cameron Stauth, *The False Fat Diet: The Revolutionary 21-Day Program for Losing the Weight You Think Is Fat* (New York: Ballantine Books, 2000).

28. Brenda Watson, *Gut Solutions: Natural Solutions for Your Digestive Conditions* (Clearwater, FL: Renew Life Press, 2003), 79.

29. Qing Yang, "Gain Weight by 'Going Diet?' Artificial Sweeteners and the Neurobiology of Sugar Cravings: Neuroscience 2010," *The Yale Journal of Biology and Medicine* 83, no. 2 (June 2010): 101–108, https://www.ncbi.nlm.nih.gov/pmc/articles/PMC2892765/.

30. Dr. Gail Matthews, "Goals Research Summary," research on goal-setting, Dominican University website, accessed December 15, 2016, http://www.dominican.edu/academics/ahss/undergraduate-programs/psych/faculty/assets-gail-matthews/researchsummary2.pdf.

31. Gretchen Rubin, *Better than Before: What I Learned about Making and Breaking Habits* (New York: Penguin Random House, 2015): 192–93.

32. David R. Hawkins, *Power vs. Force: The Hidden Determinants of Human Behavior* (Carlsbad, CA: Hay House, Inc., 2002): 91, 99–100, 260.

33. Hudnall and Kratina, *Disordered Eating*, 44.

34. "Insufficient Sleep Is a Public Health Problem," Centers for Disease Control and Prevention, September 3, 2015, accessed December 15, 2016, https://www.cdc.gov/features/dssleep.

35. Rubin, *Better than Before*.

36. Hawkins, *Power vs. Force*.

37. T. Harv Eker, "Stop Waiting to Manage Your Money... The Habit Is More Important than the Amount," on T. Harv Eker's website, accessed December 15, 2016, http://www.harveker.com/2015/09/22/stop-waiting-to-manage-your-money-the-habit-is-more-important-than-the-amount.

38. "Cheat," *The Concise Oxford Dictionary*, 9th edition (London: Oxford University Press, 1995): 223.

39. Rodika Tchi, "Easy Clutter Clearing with Feng Shui: The Best System EVER," about home, March 30, 2016, accessed December 15, 2016, http://fengshui.about.com/od/clearyourcluttertips/ss/feng-shui-clutter-clearing-system-prepare.htm.

Food, Fitness, and Sleep Tracker (with Hunger Homework): www.FindingYourForeverBody.com/Resources

Nutrition Resource: www.FindingYourForeverBody.com/Resources

Self-Talk Detox guided body-love meditation: www.FindingYourForeverBody.com/Resources

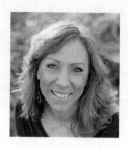

About the Author

· · · · ·

KIMBERLEY RECORD is a Registered Holistic Nutritionist (RHN) and Body Love Coach. She loves food and
the pleasure of eating, hasn't touched a diet book in more
than ten years and is proud to say she has no idea how much
she weighs. But it wasn't always that way. After many years
of body-weight obsession, calorie-counting and a relent-
less focus on her imperfections, she realized there's no
such thing as the perfect body, and the only way to truly
love our bodies is to first love who we are. This was the first
step on a life-changing journey of self-discovery based on
nutrition, fitness, and good mental, emotional and spiritual
health. Today, she knows her body is her vehicle, not her
identity, and she has developed the "Body Love toolbox"
to help separate body size from self-worth. Find out more
about creating, sharpening and maximizing your own tools
at KimberleyRecord.com. Kimberley lives on Vancouver
Island with her partner and daughter.

Get the Most of Your Forever Body Journey

. . . .

You don't have to do this alone!

. . . .

Take advantage of the supplemental resources and support available at your fingertips by visiting:

1. **www.FindingYourForeverBody.com/Resources**

   To access your free *Online Nutrition Resource; Food, Fitness, and Sleep Tracker* PDF*;* and *Self-Talk Detox* MP3 (with BONUS Body Love journal).

2. **www.KimberleyRecord.com**

   For more Body Love tips, tools, and resources; to contact Kimberley for coaching, speaking, or other inquiries; or to simply connect!

. . . .

"When you shine your gifts, you define your beauty."
KIMBERLEY RECORD